"A masterpiece of a roadmap designed to bring love, acceptance, freedom, and, most of all, balance back into the lives of those torn up by the claws of addictions."

—LINDSAY ROBERTS, Author, speaker, and co-host of *The Place for Miracles* and host of *Make Your Day Count*

"Dr. Rhona has the unique and potent combination of her personal recovery experience as well as professional training to help those still suffering. Her book brings to life what food addiction is, the research that substantiates it, and hope for anyone still suffering. There is a way to freedom!"

—KIM DENNIS, MD, CEDS, CEO and Medical Director, Timberline Knolls

"As someone who struggled most of my life with food, I wish I could have given this book to myself years ago!"

—MICHELLE AGUILAR, Author of *Becoming Fearless* and Season 6 winner of *The Biggest Loser*

Satisfied

Satisfied

A 90-DAY
SPIRITUAL JOURNEY TOWARD
Food Freedom

Dr. RHONA EPSTEIN, Psy.D
CERTIFIED ADDICTIONS COUNSELOR

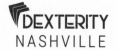
DEXTERITY
NASHVILLE

Dexterity, LLC
604 Magnolia Lane
Nashville, TN 37211
Copyright © 2018

First Edition: 2017

10 9 8 7 6 5 4 3

Printed in the United States of America

For anyone who has the courage to face his or her food problem,
I dedicate this book to you.

May you find God's strength to overcome your weakness.

For He has satisfied the thirsty soul, and the hungry soul He has filled with what is good.

PSALM 107:9 NASB

Table of Contents

SECTION TWO: SOUL-HEALING

SECTION THREE: LIVING IN FREEDOM, ONE DAY AT A TIME

INTRODUCTION

I know the deep courage it may have required to pick up this devotional. As you read these words, I want you to understand how brave you are in taking this very first step toward freedom. I haven't just studied food addiction and recovery; I have lived through it and overcome it. I know all about the struggle to put one foot in front of the other, one step at a time, toward a life of freedom. I remember the lost hope, the depressing cycle of one failed diet after another, and the inevitability of serious health problems.

I, too, was once in an oppressive, unhealthy relationship with food. Yes, I ate half-gallons of rocky road ice cream, entire boxes of Double Stuf Oreos, and jars of peanut butter while pretending to everyone (including myself) that I was on a restrictive diet. I exercised like a fanatic. I took pills to lose weight. I tried *every* gimmick on the market to control my eating, and I failed . . . over and over and over again.

I didn't understand that sugar is more addictive than cocaine.

I didn't know that the very wiring of my brain made me more vulnerable to food abuse.

I didn't realize that food calmed my nerves, much like sedatives soothing angry feelings and lifting sad ones. I didn't recognize that bingeing was my great escape from reality.

I didn't understand that my addiction was physical, emotional, and *spiritual*.

I wanted *desperately* to be healthy, but the food—the sugar—had me, and I couldn't escape its grip.

My self-esteem was destroyed. I hated myself for not being able to stay on a diet.

My relationships suffered. I slowly pulled away from people, convincing myself that my friends and family felt the same disdain for me that I felt inside. My work suffered. And yes, at my lowest point, I even began to fantasize about checking out of life.

I had lost hope that anything could change. And then the miracle happened: I found help . . . and it was NOT a diet.

The slow and steady transformation of my mind, my body, and most importantly, my soul—one small step at a time—led me into the lasting freedom promised by the only One truly able to satisfy the longings of my aching heart and soul. It was a journey that began with the knowledge, wisdom, and grace found in the pages ahead. I want to encourage you that if I can do it, you certainly can too!

Hope is found in each footstep forward . . .

I want to invite you to take your first bold steps toward freedom. I want to help transform the way you relate to food, so that it takes its proper place in your life. This struggle is equal parts physical, mental, and spiritual. I hope to equip you with practical and time-tested strategies and tools, as well as the spiritual direction, essential to your journey toward freedom from food abuse.

As a follower of Jesus, I believe the path toward transformation begins with your *soul*, so let's take our first steps together with a prayer:

I pray that God will empower you to find liberty from food abuse and addiction through His truth. I pray that you will no longer be held captive by obsessive thoughts about food or your unhealthy views of the body God gave you. May the Lord be your strength in your weakness. May you find yourself in a new relationship with Him in which you experience His love in a deeper way than you ever could have imagined. May you truly be filled with the Spirit and no longer held in chains. I pray that you will feel the presence of God surrounding you, encouraging you, and holding your hand in every step forward. And may God use your transformation to bring freedom into the lives of others. Amen.

In His hope,

Dr. Rhona

HOW TO MAKE THE MOST
OF THIS DEVOTIONAL

To change your mind, heart, and attitude, you must give your full attention to this process. Don't take this lightly. Allow yourself the gift of time and energy to care about your life and love yourself back to health.

I promise that, though it may not be easy, it will be worth it!

Give yourself ninety days to focus your attention on your recovery.

And make it the most *important* part of your day—every day.

Other Suggestions

1. Find a support group that understands overcoming overeating and food addiction.

2. Develop a healthy, satisfying food plan that eliminates all foods of abuse, including sugar and refined carbohydrates (A nutritionist would be helpful for this step).

3. Be sure your food plan is structured and clear. Don't eat outside the boundaries of what you plan unless necessary, and then ask for help with how to make needed changes. Learn to plan what you eat and eat what you plan. Practice

living with routine and structure. Doing so works better for people who have lost control.

4. Create an accountability circle of at least five people you can call on for support.

5. Don't rush through the devotional readings. Take your time and think about how each message relates to you. Write down your thoughts and reactions.

6. Every devotion ends with a "Freedom Reflection" activity. Each activity represents one step toward freedom! Complete the exercises and share them with someone you trust.

7. If you miss a day, don't worry. You can take whatever time you need. Don't give up!

This book is organized into three sections, which are influenced by the twelve steps of Alcoholics Anonymous and Overeaters Anonymous. Yet they are also deeply grounded in the spiritual truths of the Bible.

Section one addresses the honesty required to face your food problem. We examine the importance of admitting you need help and finding a spiritual solution.

Section two focuses more on underlying issues of food abuse—the emotional and relational triggers and the challenging character issues. Each day's devotional includes God-infused hope and encouragement, so try not to be afraid as you dive into these days. You will be challenged, but you will also be blessed as you discover God's strength to help you through each message.

Section three covers a broader range of practical skills and ideas to help you sustain long-term change, such as: how to manage daily life challenges without food abuse; how to handle emotional triggers; how to keep close to God for the provision of spiritual sustenance (filling the void that food once filled); and how to deal with temptation and relapse.

Finally, remember to be patient with yourself! Your problem with food did not develop overnight, and the solution will take some time to work through. If you approach this process one step at a time—one day at a time—you can discover and experience lasting freedom!

* *Throughout this devotional you will find terms such as: food addiction, addiction, recovery, food abuse, food addict, addict, overeating, overeater, and excessive eating. While you may not identify as a food addict, you may relate to some of the symptoms. This book is written for you if you are in a challenging relationship with food at any level—from the occasional loss of control to full-blown food addiction.*

Section One

HELP! I'M STUCK!

I do not understand what I do. For what I want to do I do not do, but what I hate I do. And if I do what I do not want to do, I agree that the law is good. As it is, it is no longer I myself who do it, but it is sin living in me. For I know that good itself does not dwell in me, that is, in my sinful nature. For I have the desire to do what is good, but I cannot carry it out. For I do not do the good I want to do, but the evil I do not want to do—this I keep on doing. Now if I do what I do not want to do, it is no longer I who do it, but it is sin living in me that does it.

So I find this law at work: Although I want to do good, evil is right there with me. For in my inner being I delight in God's law; but I see another law at work in me, waging war against the law of my mind and making me a prisoner of the law of sin at work within me. What a wretched man I am! Who will rescue me from this body that is subject to death? Thanks be to God, who delivers me through Jesus Christ our Lord!

ROMANS 7:15–25 NIV

Day 1

Let's Begin by Being Honest

I do not understand what I do.
For what I want to do I do not do, but what I hate I do.
ROMANS 7:15 NIV

❧

Anyone who struggles with an addiction can identify with thoughts like: *What is wrong with me? I should know better! Why can't I just stop overeating?* I remember saying these words to myself each day. It is comforting to discover the same feelings in the Bible from a faithful man of God. Like us, Paul was keenly aware of his own internal battle and didn't understand why he couldn't just "do what is right" either! But in this scripture, Paul is also modeling the type of ruthless honesty that is a necessary starting point for change.

It isn't easy to come to terms with the reality that *everything* you've tried has failed, but it is the very place where God can begin working in your life. If you want to take your first step toward healing, you must begin with the admission that your way is simply not working. It's time to accept that you need help!

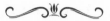

If you want to take your first step toward healing, you must begin with the admission that your way is simply not working.

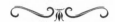

Freedom Reflection

I'd like you to list all of the diets you have tried and the results of each one (Go ahead and write out the whole story— the temporary successes, the failures, all of it.). Do you wake up promising yourself today will be different, only to end up in the same mess tomorrow? Be honest. How much money do you spend on binges and fad diets? How much time and energy goes into the process of fighting your food addiction? Is it really working?

Day 2

Yes, I Am Full of Despair

I am worn out from sobbing. All night I flood my bed with weeping, drenching it with my tears. My vision is blurred by grief; my eyes are worn out because of all my enemies.

PSALM 6:6–7

It is so important to begin with the admission that you are spiritually and emotionally exhausted from this battle with food abuse, but also to understand that you are physically worn out because the food itself makes you feel ill. Sugar causes you to become depressed, moody, and lethargic, and your excess weight may be affecting your quality of life!

Be honest with yourself: You know in your heart that you are out of control, and this causes you deep sorrow.

The heaviness of your addiction is always present in pain, sadness, and hopelessness. The despair of the Psalmist is also your despair. Yet it is in these very psalms that you can discover the power in being honest with yourself and the God who loves you.

Freedom Reflection

Write about how you *really* feel about your eating, weight, and body image. What do you think about what is happening in your life? Be thorough and honest. Before we can focus on solutions, we must face our true feelings about this problem.

Day 3

It's Okay to Say, "I Don't Know"

Anyone who claims to know all the answers
doesn't really know very much.

1 CORINTHIANS 8:2

I understand that you may have learned how to eat better or lose weight. You might know enough to teach classes on nutrition and behavior modification. You may even have schooling on the topic like I do, but that knowledge will not solve your problem. If you are going to really change, you need to become teachable!

Today, I want you to allow yourself to simply say, "I don't know." I want you to become a student again. Learn to be curious. Be open to new ideas! Some of what you've already learned will come in handy, but don't hold on to the idea that you have all the answers. With that attitude, you might just miss the help

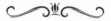

If you are going to really change, you need to become teachable!

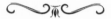

you need! This is your time to learn and grow, and that can only happen when you are open and humble.

Freedom Reflection

Spend some time writing about how it feels to let yourself be teachable, especially when you already have a head full of knowledge. In what areas do you struggle with a know-it-all attitude? How might that hinder you from getting all you can out of this process?

Day 4

Am I Addicted to Sugar?

For you have been called to live in freedom.
GALATIANS 5:13

❧

Did you know that science has only recently discovered that sugar is an addictive substance? Dr. Mark Hyman, author of *Eat Fat, Get Thin*, writes, "Sugar and processed foods have been shown to be eight times more addictive than cocaine."[1] Scientists can now actually identify the difference between people who have sugar addictions and those who don't by simply looking at brain scans! I'm willing to bet that you had no idea when you first enjoyed a sugary treat that you were indulging in a behavior that could ruin your life. Society, family, and friends have all told you sugar was good, fun, and enjoyable; and on top of that, it is readily available *everywhere* you look. No one warned you about the possible addiction, the way they did with cigarettes, drugs, and alcohol. You didn't know the risk! To be fair, no one knew until recently.

You are different from other people in the way you relate to food. You understand it isn't normal to hide, sneak, and lie about what you eat. The truth is, you have a problem; it's *not* normal to think about food all day long and to make meals and snacks the focal points of your day.

Freedom Reflection

Be honest about your daily habits: Are you addicted to sugar? Do you consistently eat more than you intend? Do you ever eat until you become sick? Do you eat large quantities? Do you crave it? Do you eat for emotional reasons? What other foods may you be addicted to?

Day 5

Make These Cravings Stop!

The spirit is willing, but the flesh is weak.
MATTHEW 26:41 NIV

We have to understand *the forces* we are fighting against if we are going to make lasting progress. Science now tells us that there is a deep connection between sugar and uncontrollable cravings. In fact, sugar actually hijacks your brain and makes you addicted! Dopamine, the "feel-good" chemical in your brain, becomes overstimulated when you eat too much sugar. And when that happens, you need more and more to get—and to sustain—those good feelings. The cravings eventually become unmanageable. You see, that drive is *biological*, and until you detox your body from sugar, those sugar-induced cravings will be an obstacle for following *any* sort of healthy eating plan![2]

Now that you understand you are in a battle with a *physiological* addiction, you can better equip yourself to overcome it (Remember that sugar is actually hidden in many of the foods we eat, and refined carbohydrates have the same effect that sugar does on the body)!

Freedom Reflection

Go through your kitchen and examine the labels on the foods you eat. What are the ingredients (Go online to find a list of all the names for sugar so you know what to look for)?

The ingredients in what you eat are always listed in order from most to least. If sugar is past the fifth ingredient on the list, the item probably doesn't contain enough sugar to "trip" the addiction wire. Make a habit of reading labels in the grocery store, too. There is power in better understanding what you are putting into your body. Most processed foods are loaded with sugar—including the ones that claim to be "health" or "diet foods." Write down what you learn from reading your labels.

Day 6

Let Go of Self-Condemnation

So now there is no condemnation
for those who belong to Christ Jesus.

Romans 8:1

Let's be honest. You would *never* allow someone to speak to a family member or a loved one the way you talk to yourself! If you are a parent, what would you do if you overheard someone speaking to your child with that kind of negativity? Maybe it is time to remember that you are God's child. I pray that you will hear this truth today: You've beaten yourself up long enough! All of this negative self-talk is destructive. It is time to accept some grace. You didn't know the sweets you enjoyed as a child were more addictive than cocaine! You didn't know when you turned to food for stress relief or comfort that you could become hooked. You may not have become overweight and imprisoned by addiction if you could have avoided it!

My prayer for you is to realize that you are forgiven. God holds nothing against you: He wants you to stop beating yourself up and start trusting in His forgiveness and grace! The discouragement that follows your negative self-talk will only lead you back to needing food for relief. Instead, I want you to remember the truth: You are a child of God. You are not condemned. You are forgiven. Today, I hope you will begin to embrace that unconditional love!

Freedom Reflection

Take time to research and write a list of scriptures that affirm God's unconditional love for you, and then meditate on them today (It is even helpful to memorize a few of them and recite them whenever you begin to think badly about yourself!). Spend some time writing down what these verses mean to you, and how the truth of God's love can help you let go of negativity and food addiction.

Day 7

Finding Strength in Your Weakness

That's why I take pleasure in my weaknesses, and in the insults, hardships, persecutions, and troubles that I suffer for Christ. For when I am weak, then I am strong.

2 CORINTHIANS 12:10

I know it is not easy to admit weakness. Some days, the simple acknowledgment that you need help can be so difficult! In our "have it all together" culture, admitting you need help can be terrifying. Maybe you feel that no one will understand your food addiction. You imagine them saying, "Just eat better and exercise. Simple, right?"

I believe it is empowering to take Paul's approach and learn to "take pleasure" in your weakness. Admitting your own weakness opens the door for God to come into your broken places and bring strength. When you let yourself be honest and

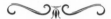

Admitting your own weakness opens the door
for God to come into your broken places
and bring strength.

broken before Him, you can then invite Him to help—and He
is able to do far better things than you can imagine.

It may not make sense to take pleasure in your weakness. It
goes against all you've ever learned about being strong and fighting
the good fight, but this is the day to let Him be your strength.

Freedom Reflection

Write what the words in this verse mean to you: *For when
I am weak, then I am strong.* How does this Biblical truth apply
to your recovery and healing from food addiction?

Day 8

Admitting You Are Powerless

When we were utterly helpless,
Christ came at just the right time and died for us.
ROMANS 5:6

The first step of the Overeaters Anonymous twelve-step program is simple: "We admitted we were powerless over food—that our lives had become unmanageable."[3] I understand that you have tried hard enough to fight this problem on your own, but your attempts at control have only led you into despair and discouragement. Maybe you feel as though you have hit bottom. You may even be wondering, *How much worse does it need to get before I get better?*

I know the admission of your own powerlessness before addiction can feel like defeat in the moment, but it is actually a resounding victory! Throughout the Bible, the admission of powerlessness by God's children is the very thing that launches Him into action. Once you are at a place of admitting you can't end this eating addiction on your own, then you are ready for His divine power to enter, transform your life, and take you to places you never could have imagined. Remember: with you alone, this fight is impossible. But with God, all things are possible!

Freedom Reflection

Spend a few moments writing about what "powerlessness" means to you. What does it feel like? What is "hitting rock bottom" like for you regarding your eating and obsession with food and weight? In what areas has your life become unmanageable?

Day 9

What's Really Holding You Back?

Therefore, since we are surrounded by such a huge crowd of witnesses to the life of faith, let us strip off every weight that slows us down, especially the sin that so easily trips us up. And let us run with endurance the race God has set before us.

HEBREWS 12:1

I know you've thought about fixing your eating problem and considered the alternatives. You may have attempted this many times before and failed. I want you to see those attempts—and those failures—as lessons. When you've been caught in addiction for so long, it takes time and effort for new behaviors and attitudes to stick.

Lasting change is a *process*. It *only* happens one day at a time, by putting one foot in front of the other. Yes, setbacks and challenges are going to come, and they will make you feel like quitting; but when they do, I challenge you to pick yourself up and take another step forward. Each day that you stick with your plan and use your support is one more step toward becoming the new you!

Freedom Reflection

What do you think is hindering you from sticking with healthy eating? Do you become impatient with the process and give up too easily? Do you become bored or lazy about planning and preparing? Do social pressures cause you to give up on your goals? Write a list of the hindrances to your recovery. What can you do to get past them?

Day 10

Are You Ready?

When Jesus saw him and knew he had been ill for a long time, he asked him, "Would you like to get well?"

JOHN 5:6

You already know you *need* to get well. You understand that you *should* be ready for all that God has for you. You are well aware that you'd be so much happier if you ate healthy food and if your body were in better condition. As Christians, we understand that healing begins with admitting our problem and calling out to God for help. Of course, it begins by saying *yes* to Jesus: *Yes! I want to get well!*

Why do you still hesitate? Because of the addiction! Even though you want to be free from the pain, the weight, and the insanity, you really don't want to live without the comfort food brings from stress and anxiety. Food gives you something, and though it comes with grave consequences, you like the pleasure of a good binge. The excess food is there for a reason . . .

My friend, now that you understand how Jesus has personally invited you into divine healing, you may ask: "Am I *really* ready for this?"

Freedom Reflection

Spend some time today prayerfully considering these questions: Are you ready to invite Jesus to participate in your journey from addiction to freedom? What does your food addiction give you that you cannot let go of? Why might you want to keep it around? Imagine life without your addiction, then imagine all of the obstacles in the way of that life. Spend some time in prayer over each item on that list.

Day 11

You Can Talk to God As You Are, Right Where You Are

*And I am convinced that nothing
can ever separate us from God's love.*
ROMANS 8:38

Today, I want to remind you that God is not "out there" waiting on you: He will meet you right where you are—just as you are—if you'll just reach out for Him.

You might be feeling some hesitation about changing your eating habits and giving up your favorite foods (even if they are killing you)! Rest assured: God will show up where you are even if everything inside you is screaming, *No way! I like my sweets and my all-you-can-eat buffet meals way too much. I don't want to change!*

You may feel completely prepared to leave addiction behind. If you are ready, make sure to talk to God about how much you need Him to help—because your way doesn't work! You may even need to ask forgiveness for forgetting about Him amid your previous attempts to fix your problem. Ask Him for the faith to depend on His strength.

No matter where your heart is along this journey, know that He will show up and enable you to do what you could not do before.

Ask Him for the faith to depend on His strength.

Freedom Reflection

I want to challenge you to talk to God honestly about *everything* you are thinking and feeling about your struggle with food addiction. Talk to Him whether you are feeling defeated by addiction or ready and willing to change. Most importantly, open your mind and heart to listen. Remember: God loves you no matter what!

Day 12

Lord, Please Help My Unbelief

I do believe, but help me overcome my unbelief!
MARK 9:24

∾

It is difficult to believe you can finally be well when you have messed up so many times. But today, I want you to be honest about whether you have truly sought God's help and strength in this battle with addiction. Have you ever invited Him to participate in this journey with you—or has this been your own fight? Your own strength fails, but God's never does.

It's a whole different story when you learn to depend on God. Do you truly believe He wants you to be free from food dependency? Do you know that He sees you in your struggles and He longs for you to walk in freedom? Jesus came to break chains and set you free. He came for you. He is here for you and is ready to help.

Freedom Reflection

How do you relate to the verse above? Write about your struggle with doubt and how it hinders you from going to God with your addiction. Are you ready to ask God to help your unbelief? Don't wait any longer! Ask and He will deliver!

Day 13

If You Fail to Plan, Then You Plan to Fail

But the Holy Spirit produces . . . self-control.
GALATIANS 5:22–23

❧

As you begin your freedom journey, one of the toughest challenges is food planning. You may resist the idea of shopping for healthier foods, of going through the trouble of preparing and packing meals, and of taking the time and care to make sure the quantities are correct. My friend, discipline is not easy!

Recovery rarely happens without planning.

It is way too easy to fall back into bad habits, like eating unhealthy meals when you have no plan in place. It's important to set aside time each week—each day—to make clear and determined plans. Knowing what foods and eating behaviors you need to avoid is just the beginning. It also helps to have accountability in the early days of change to help you get on track.

Freedom Reflection

Are you fighting against the idea of a food plan, or are you embracing the discipline of a clear plan for eating? Write honestly about where you are in this process. Food planning can remove confusion and bring peace to your mealtime. Are you ready to take the necessary steps to build a plan and stick to it? Why or why not?

Day 14

You Can't Do This Alone!

Plans go wrong for lack of advice; many advisers bring success.
PROVERBS 15:22

Finding the right support is a necessary part of getting started in this process. I understand that it may be one of the things holding you back. Food is a central part of living, and as you set out toward freedom, you will quickly realize how entangled this problem is in almost every area of your day.

If you are resistant to letting people help you, it's a good time to challenge that. You see, most people don't recover alone. In fact, the Bible tells us that we weren't meant to do anything significant on our own. We really do need the help of others, especially since addiction is mainly a problem of *isolation*. Our destructive eating is often done in secret. Our shame is experienced privately.

True power lies in reaching out to those who have experienced the same addiction, who have walked ahead of you on the road to recovery. Leaning into a community actually helps alleviate your shame. There are so many people who have been on the same journey, and they can be a great source of strength and encouragement. They can help you when you slip up and make you feel less alone on your road to freedom!

Freedom Reflection

How do you feel about letting people help you with your eating issues? Are you willing to be real and vulnerable with others so you can receive the strength, encouragement, and spiritual guidance you need? Write down a list of groups, professionals, friends, or family whom you would trust to walk with you on your road to recovery.

Day 15

Happiness Is an Inside Job

Though our outer man is decaying, yet our inner man is being renewed day by day. For momentary, light affliction is producing for us an eternal weight of glory far beyond all comparison.
2 CORINTHIANS 4:16–17 NASB

Today's culture bombards you with advertisements. In almost every form of media, marketers take aim at your looks. Everything is about *appearance*: your weight, skin, makeup, or hair. Of course, there is nothing wrong with wanting to look good on the outside—as long as you truly understand the shallowness, the spiritual bankruptcy, and the fallacy of our culture's ideas about beauty and perfection. Your journey is toward a healthy body and soul! The Bible tells us that our heart is what matters most.

If your heart is right, it will make all the difference in how you feel about your life. Practice being more concerned about closeness to God, hearing His voice, knowing Him, trusting Him to satisfy you, and finding His peace. Remember that lasting change in every area of your life happens when you focus on the work of the Holy Spirit within you. Make it a goal to prioritize Jesus. His Spirit will shine through better than anything you can find in the beauty aisle.

Freedom Reflection

Describe how you see people who walk closely with God. Can you see the glow and the touch of heaven on them? How does that compare to beauty products or the fake messages about youth and perfection we see in advertising?

Day 16

Focus on the Solution
Rather Than the Problem

*And you will know the truth,
and the truth will set you free.*
JOHN 8:32

It's easy to get caught up in worrying about how to get out of this addiction. You can become obsessively focused on the extra pounds, the bingeing, and the self-hatred, and doing so can make you depressed. I want to challenge you to stop focusing on the problems and to begin developing a solution-focused mindset!

I know this can feel overwhelming. Your mind will want to return, over and over again, to worry. But focus on the truth that you are a new creation. God promises that you are free and that there is always a way of escaping temptation. The truth *will* set you free. Be determined to practice believing. The power of God is stronger than the power of the addiction! Yes, the addiction may feel stronger than you at times, but it is no match for the Lord.

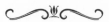

The power of God is stronger than the power of the addiction!

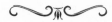

Freedom Reflection

Take time to repeat the truth to yourself throughout the day: *The Lord has set me free!*

Day 17

The Power of God Is in Me

Indeed, we felt we had received the sentence of death.
But this happened that we might not rely on
ourselves but on God, who raises the dead.

2 CORINTHIANS 1:9 NIV

You are here because you have been beaten down by overeating, food abuse, and weight obsession. It has taken everything from you. Addiction has stolen your hope. You have hit bottom and know the only path to real change is through spiritual transformation—a miracle—a God-given gift of freedom.

I promise you that when you come to trust the Lord with your problems, you can accomplish what was impossible in your own strength. Victory begins when you believe in the One with the power to resurrect the parts of you that died in addiction. The hope for freedom is only found in the power of the omnipotent, loving God inside you—the God who satisfies your every need.

Freedom Reflection

Write about the difference between trusting yourself and depending on God. What does it mean to you to have the power of God who raises the dead inside you? Do you believe in that power? List the reasons why and remind yourself throughout the day.

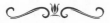

Victory begins when you believe
in the One with the power to resurrect the
parts of you that died in addiction.

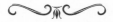

Day 18

I Can't, but He Can . . . So I'll Let Him

Not that we are adequate in ourselves to consider anything
as coming from ourselves, but our adequacy is from God.
2 Corinthians 3:5 NASB

In theory, it may be easy to recognize your inadequacy without God, but in day-to-day practice, it is difficult to give control to Him. If you are like me, you are often tempted to rely on your own strength, even when you know it will lead to failure and disappointment! If you feel defeated, take a moment and pay attention to the truth found in today's verse. I challenge you to learn what it really means to live it out in your daily life.

When you understand that your adequacy comes from God, you will approach challenges differently. You will hold on to God, knowing your success comes from your relationship with Him. Complete dependence on God is never easy, but it's necessary. The Bible is filled with stories of people just like you and me who did great things because they learned to depend on God. Being honest about our own inadequacy and our reliance on God is truly the hope for our victory.

Freedom Reflection

Write about the strength that comes from realizing you don't have to be adequate by yourself. Explain why it's okay to be imperfect and to not have it all together. Write a prayer inviting the Lord into your inadequacies today.

Day 19

All Things New

Therefore if anyone is in Christ, he is a new creature; the old things passed away; behold, new things have come.

2 Corinthians 5:17 NASB

If you ponder this verse and believe what the scripture says, you understand that when you became a believer you actually became a new person. It can be difficult to see this truth when you cling to old, unhealthy views and behaviors. How can you feel new when you just see the same old, addicted, obsessed person?

By faith, I want to challenge you to actually take hold of this truth about renewal. Meditate on today's scripture, and know that the prison doors of your addiction have been unlocked by Jesus. You are not a prisoner anymore; you are free! You are a new creation in Christ! You now have the power of God in you to rise above temptation, lies, and defeat. You have the power to live a life of victory.

Freedom Reflection

Spend some time writing about what these words mean to you today: "Old things passed away; behold, new things have come." How does this relate to your recovery? What old things do you need to let pass away today? Describe who you are as a new creation.

Day 20

Choose God First!

Let us purify ourselves from everything that contaminates body and spirit, perfecting holiness out of reverence.

2 Corinthians 7:1 niv

Purifying yourself from unhealthy eating is a necessary step in your healing journey. I know from experience that ridding your life of junk food and unhealthy dietary choices can be a challenge. There will be temptations at every turn, but let the Biblical idea of purification inspire you toward your goal. Junk and excess, in any form, can be blocks to holiness, so choose the better path and let them go!

Make the decision for holiness in all you do. Choose God! Don't fool yourself into thinking that you can have it both ways. The darkness that comes with food abuse will dull the sweetness of the life God has designed you to live. Today, focus on leaving

~~~ ⚜ ~~~

Make the decision for holiness in all you do.

~~~ ⚜ ~~~

the unhealthy use of food as a means of drawing closer to God, and watch the light of His love begin to wipe out the darkness of addiction!

Freedom Reflection

What are you hanging onto in your eating and behavior that is contaminating you and keeping you from experiencing all God desires for you? Write it down and ask for help letting go of anything impure.

Day 21

Love the Body God Gave You

No one hates his own body but feeds and cares for it.
EPHESIANS 5:29

Part of loving yourself involves loving your own body. The Bible tells us that your body is a temple for the Holy Spirit, so let's be really honest: No one who loves their own body abuses it with amounts of junk food that cause obesity, diabetes, skin problems, heart disease, etc. No one who loves their body puts it through cycles of starvation and bingeing. Loving your body means caring for yourself by eating healthy foods and exercising.

Of course, it takes time, effort, and intention to care for your body. There are endless excuses: you may feel you are too busy, or maybe you don't like healthy food. But in your heart, you know that your excuses are unacceptable. You are responsible to care for the body God gave you.

I want you to begin to think of yourself as you would a friend. How would you treat a friend? Would you abuse your friend? Would you only feed your friend junk food? Would you starve your friend for punishment? Of course you wouldn't! It is time to give your body the same consideration.

Freedom Reflection

First, write a letter of apology to yourself for the ways you have abused your body. In the letter, promise to treat your body with love and respect. Then write out a plan to put that resolution into practice.

Day 22

Living Free from the Pit

He lifted me out of the pit of despair, out of the mud and the mire.
He set my feet on solid ground and steadied me as I walked along.

PSALM 40:2

∽

It is not far-fetched to say that food addiction is a pit of despair. I know from experience that it is a terrible feeling to be caught in such bondage. Addiction causes loneliness and isolation; but the Bible tells us that God is merciful and good. He can lift you up, put you on solid ground, and help you walk steady. God can enable you to live free of despair.

Many people grow hopeless and resign themselves to living day to day in the pit of despair. Why? Because after so many years—no matter how hopeless and painful—it becomes a familiar living space. If you have been there long enough, you may even forget what life outside of that pit looks like.

Today, let's fight despair by giving thanks! God has promised you a way out of this addiction. In prayer, reach for His hand and let Him pull you out of your daily life of hopelessness. Take hold of the support He provides, ask for courage to climb out of the daily despair, take His hand, and let Him lead you toward freedom.

Today, let's fight despair
by giving thanks!

Freedom Reflection

What are some habits and ways of thinking that can lead you back into the familiar pit? What are some practical steps that can help you resist revisiting despair?

Day 23

All Things Are Possible with God

Humanly speaking, it is impossible.
But with God everything is possible.

MATTHEW 19:26

I believe that some verses are worth repeating several times a day. When you are working to make a difficult but necessary life change, repeating a scripture can provide inner strength. Daily, I hope you will remind yourself that everything is possible with God. That simple truth will carry you through the challenges of every meal and every temptation. It's easy to feel defeated after years of proven failure, but you are on a new journey where you are learning to trust God with your recovery.

As you go about your day, remember to invite God into every moment. Set alarms on your phone or put notes around the house to remind yourself to rely on God in all things. You were vulnerable to overeating because you convinced yourself that food could fulfill what only God can, but if you turn to God to meet your needs, you will truly be filled. Alone you were hopeless, but with Him, all things are possible!

Freedom Reflection

Create reminders to pray and cues to stay focused on the verses you are learning each day. Write down faith-building verses on sticky notes and put them around your home and office, where you can be reminded to trust God, pray, and believe!

Day 24

An Overflowing Hope

---

*May the God of hope fill you with all joy and peace
as you trust in him, so that you may overflow with hope
by the power of the Holy Spirit.*

ROMANS 15:13 NIV

It's difficult to maintain hope sometimes, especially when things have not been going well. I remember the moments in my own recovery when I could barely imagine moving forward. But hope is like oxygen to our journey to freedom from addiction! In your moments of hopelessness, remember this Scripture: *"May the God of hope* [just those words can start to spark hope into your soul] *fill you will all joy and peace as you trust in him* [this is our part; we need to trust Him], *so that you may overflow with hope by the power of the Holy Spirit."*

Today, I challenge you to memorize Romans 15:13 as your reminder to hope in God for your transformation. Our hope on this journey to recovery is in Him, that He will break the chains of food addiction or food abuse. If you can make it a way of life to meditate on His overflowing hope, you will be amazed by what the Lord will do in your life.

Freedom Reflection

Imagine living your life in hope—filled with joy, peace, and trust in God. Imagine that your hope was overflowing with the power of the Holy Spirit. Write down what you believe your life could be like.

Day 25

Praise Him in the Battle

I call upon the Lord, who is worthy to be praised,
And I am saved from my enemies.

PSALM 18:3 NASB

Recovering from an addiction can often feel like a full-on battle. You can get motivated and ready for a good day, say your prayers, and read encouraging, inspirational readings; but before you know it, temptations are aggressively knocking at your door.

Especially in the beginning stages of recovery, you will feel as though you are constantly fighting destructive urges off the doorstep. Eventually, though, the force behind your addiction—yes, the enemy—will realize that you mean business. Don't be afraid or discouraged by these onslaughts of temptation. Fighting them off is part of the process.

It is empowering to understand temptations. Some are physiological cravings, some are habit, some are emotional, and some are truly of the devil. Be prepared for them to show up. Expect the fight to come, and be determined to answer back with a clear commitment to your recovery. Keep slamming the door on temptation until it stays out. And remember: you must keep the door to all addictive behaviors sealed shut if you want those temptations to stop. Keep praying and relying on God. As the Bible tells us: Resist the devil, and he will flee!

Freedom Reflection

Do you have a favorite worship song or a powerful verse you can rely on when you feel tempted? Make a list of the songs or words that make you feel empowered by God and carry it with you in your purse or wallet. Sing, speak, or pray those words aloud whenever you need to be strengthened.

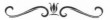

Expect the fight to come, and be determined to answer back with a clear commitment to your recovery.

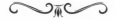

Day 26

Stand Firm on the Word of God

People do not live by bread alone,
but by every word that comes from the mouth of God.

Matthew 4:4

The Gospel of Matthew tells us that after fasting in the wilderness for forty days, Jesus was tempted by the devil. Jesus responded to these trials using the Word of God to make it clear that He would not give temptations any consideration.

During this season of breaking free from addictive eating, it's important to be steadfast and clear in your plan to combat temptation, so that when it comes you'll know exactly how to handle it. For example, if sugar is your addictive substance, you will still attend someone's birthday party on occasion. Temptation will come in a state of confusion: it may try to convince you that your rules "do not apply for birthdays." Of course, you know that your brain doesn't change on birthdays, and the addiction will reactivate if you eat cake! It's no different from an alcoholic having one drink on New Year's Eve. Once the door is opened, it could take *years* for them to sober up again.

Learning where to be clear and how to stand firm in your convictions will keep you out of trouble. Remember that Jesus had fasted for days and was hungry when the devil suggested turning the stones to bread, but He did not give in to Satan's schemes. Jesus promises that we can trust His Word for sustenance in times of trial.

Freedom Reflection

What scriptures can you lean on to help you when temptation arises? We need to learn to respond to temptation as Jesus did—by reciting Scripture and not giving in. Write down some inspirational verses and consider memorizing them to recall in difficult situations.

Day 27

It Is a Matter of Life and Death

He sent from on high, He took me;
He drew me out of many waters.

Psalm 18:16 nasb

 ∼

Abusing food feels like struggling to swim in deep waters. Addiction feels like drowning with no hope of rescue. That way of life is exhausting when you can't even see your way to shore. In Alcoholics Anonymous literature, the people who get well are referred to as those who held on to recovery principles with "all the fervor with which the drowning seize life preservers."[4]

In order to recover, it is important to always remember the sensation you had when you were drowning. Remember the feeling that led to picking up this book, going to a twelve-step meeting, attending rehab, or seeing a counselor. Recovery depends on your taking this seriously and recognizing that you could die from food addiction. Otherwise, statistics are clear that you will end up right back where you began: drowning in deep waters.

Healing is physical, emotional, and spiritual, and all aspects need to be properly addressed so you don't fall back into trouble. At some point you will feel safe. You may be tempted to believe you don't need help to get well. You must be on guard against this false sense of security. Diets alone have never worked before, so this time I encourage you to diligently pursue the complete healing of your body, mind, and spirit.

Freedom Reflection

Since diets are only short-lived, you've learned that you need a new approach. How do you understand food-addiction recovery as a body, mind, and spirit method to transformation? Be honest—are you ready for this approach, or are you still looking for a quick fix?

Day 28

You Are Touched by His Mercy

Your gentleness makes me great.
PSALM 18:35 NASB

As you move forward toward freedom, it is helpful to remember the character of the One leading you on this journey. Our Lord is gentle and kind, full of love and mercy. Jesus understands our weaknesses because He faced all of the same trials we face, and yet He did not sin (Hebrews 4:15). He would never deal with you harshly, as some may fear. Once you are reminded of His character, it's easier to approach Him as you are: broken, messy, and beaten up. Don't wait until you have it together. He accepts you just as you are.

You may hardly be able to face your weaknesses from your food battles or other character issues, but I am here to testify to the truth that God can handle all of it. He will not scold you or

56

make you feel badly for your mistakes, even if you've made them a thousand times. Today, I want you to dwell in His gentleness. I challenge you to taste His mercy and live in His grace.

Don't wait until you have
it together. He accepts you
just as you are.

Freedom Reflection

Write a letter to God telling Him how messed up you feel about your food abuse. Then, write another letter back to yourself from God, reminding yourself how you are loved unconditionally and completely forgiven.

Day 29

God's Unconditional Love

The Lord is merciful and compassionate, slow to get angry and filled with unfailing love.

PSALM 145:8

As we have discussed, shame and guilt go hand in hand with food addiction. After the binges and the awful sick feelings, the weight starts piling on, and it becomes hard to imagine anyone loving you at all. Yet God's mercy and compassion break through all that shame. You can find deep healing when you realize that God is not holding your loss of control against you. Receiving His unconditional love changes *everything* in your life.

No matter your past, you can try again because there is no shame to keep you bound. The freedom that comes from His love heals and delivers. In Jesus' parable of the prodigal son, the father celebrates the son's return without a single comment about his awful behavior. And remember how Jesus stood up for the woman who was caught in adultery? He protected her against those who wanted to stone her to death.

In the same way, our Lord forgives every single binge, every single mistake, every moment of self-loathing. He knows you have not taken care of the temple of the Holy Spirit, but He is not holding it against you. He forgives it all. And He wants you to accept His forgiveness and move on from your addictive eating into a closer walk with Him.

Freedom Reflection

Imagine yourself as the prodigal son being hugged by the father. Then imagine that you are the adulterous woman and that Jesus has not only forgiven you, but also has shielded you from those who threw stones your way. What does this say about God's feelings for you today? Write about how shame and guilt from your addictive eating may have caused you to stay away from God. Can you accept God's unconditional love for you? What is holding you back?

Day 30

It's Time to Let Others Help You

Get all the advice and instruction you can,
so you will be wise the rest of your life.
PROVERBS 19:20

Fixing your problems with food on your own hasn't worked out well. The truth is, it didn't work out well for me either when I tried it without help! Facing the fact that you need other people is a challenge I hope you will accept. Addiction is a disease of isolation and loneliness that deceives you into thinking it is safer to pick up food than it is to reach for the phone. But the comfort food once provided is a destructive force in your life, and you need other people's help to change that.

I learned early in my own recovery that God provides people who already know the way forward. God used dear friends in my journey to freedom that had walked that path and needed me to help in their own recovery.

In the coming days, I want you to gather five people in your circle who you can contact regularly for support. Choose people you know that you can count on. Make at least three contacts each day to these recovery supports in the beginning of your journey. You will find that you need different people for different aspects of your recovery. One person may provide encouragement when you need it. Someone else may provide more practical advice or assistance. Another may be good for company when you need someone to just sit next to you in silence.

And don't wait until you are in a moment of crisis to call. It is often too late by then. Relationships with recovering people will give you strength to carry on in good times and bad.

Freedom Reflection

This week, make three phone calls to people in recovery each day, just for practice. Write about your experience.

Section Two

Soul-Healing

Search me, O God, and know my heart;
test me and know my anxious thoughts.

Psalm 139:23

Day 31

Untangling Your Food and Feelings

Trust in the Lord with all your heart
and lean not on your own understanding;
in all your ways submit to him,
and he will make your paths straight.

PROVERBS 3:5 NIV

Initially, you turned to food to solve your problems—and then food *became* the problem. You didn't understand when you used food for a little soothing, a quick pick-me-up, or a break from the day that it could end up an issue of its own. You still have the original problem, but now you also carry the obsession, guilt, shame, and loss of control that come with food addiction. What a mess.

It is so important to untangle food issues from the other problems in your life. You must learn to handle life's many challenges with healthy solutions. Your struggle with food now has a life of its own, so it must be dealt with as its own separate matter. Food and your feelings must be separated. Food and coping must be separated. Food will not solve your stress, anger, loneliness, or fear. You may feel overwhelmed at this idea, but it is the truth.

Try to be patient with yourself during this process. This is a difficult step in recovery. If you have used food to cope with problems most of your life, you'll likely find yourself feeling insecure without that crutch. But if you are willing and intentional about it, you will learn new and better ways. Remember, my friend: you are not alone. The Lord is with you. Others who are on the journey and know the way can help. You can learn just as they did.

Freedom Reflection

Write about how you use food to cope with life. What are the primary areas in which you see yourself turning to food as a coping strategy?

Day 32

Change Yourself by Changing Your Mind

Let God transform you into a new person by changing the way you think. Then you will learn to know God's will for you, which is good and pleasing and perfect.

ROMANS 12:2

Let's take an honest inventory of what goes on in your mind. You have negative thoughts about food. You talk to yourself in ways you would never let anyone speak to someone you loved. You fixate on a negative body image. You obsess about your weight. You constantly worry about other people's opinions of how you look. This pattern of thinking is destructive, and it has to change! I know you desperately want to focus on your life, work, family, friends, and the Lord, but negative thoughts about food and weight keep creeping in and stealing your peace of mind.

Take courage in knowing that God can change you from the inside out. His Word tells you that He will transform you by the renewing of your mind—by actually changing the way you think. It is time to stop obsessing about your diet and condemning yourself for all your mistakes. Change the "channel" in your mind from the "negative thinking network" to something more life-giving and satisfying. Today, practice thinking about how much God loves you. Meditate on the truths found in His Word: God will never leave you nor forsake you; He will provide the strength you need to conquer this addiction. Instead of negative body-image thoughts, meditate on the truth that you are "fearfully and wonderfully made" (Psalm 139:14 NIV). Remember—you are transformed into a new person by the way you think!

Freedom Reflection

Today, make a list of five new ways you can practice thinking about yourself that would be more hopeful and transformative.

Day 33

Control What You Think

---

*We are destroying speculations and every lofty thing raised up
against the knowledge of God, and we are taking every thought
captive to the obedience of Christ.*

2 Corinthians 10:5 nasb

Your way of thinking can be a big part of your addiction,
but it can also play a huge role in your healing! You can't stop
your natural thoughts, but you can take them captive. Your
negative thoughts will always come and go. It is what you do
with them that counts. Make the decision that you will no longer
focus on or nurture negative thoughts. Yes, that is a choice you
can make, a habit you can create, and with God's help and a
commitment to change, you can become excellent at controlling
your thoughts.

Learning to master your own thoughts is a daily process that many believe is harder than physical exercise. If you remain disciplined and really work at it, you will get better at squashing negative thoughts and replacing them with truth.

It is so important to learn to recognize the thoughts related to your food addiction: the lures, temptations, and confusion that can encourage you to eat just one of those cookies when you could never eat just one before. It is also necessary to learn how to respond to these thoughts—what words to say to yourself—so you are always ready. When your mind becomes distracted, overwhelmed, or stressed, direct it back to truth and peace. Your recovery depends on keeping your mind sharp and positive. Watch over yourself and take your thoughts captive!

Freedom Reflection

Write down some of the negative thoughts you have experienced in the last few days. What did you do with them? Did you give them power, or did you capture them? How can you become more disciplined about focusing on the positive?

Day 34

Put Off the Old, and Welcome in the New

---

*Throw off your old sinful nature and your former way of life,
which is corrupted by lust and deception. Instead, let the Spirit
renew your thoughts and attitudes. Put on your new nature,
created to be like God—truly righteous and holy.*

EPHESIANS 4:22–24

By faith, you are letting go of your old, addicted self
and stepping into your new nature. It is important to examine
what you need to put aside and then what you need to put on.
Imagine getting rid of a pile of old clothing and building a new
wardrobe. You may like some of the old ways because they are
comfortable, in the same way old clothes are comfortable. We
want to hang on to negativity, resentment, avoidance, and fear,
but only because they are familiar. Food has enabled you to cover
over your real issues. It dulls you and makes you less able to see

your unresolved character issues. When you give up excess food, the character issues then must be cleaned up and thrown out, or they will keep coming back to fuel your addiction. Don't turn away from this process: God is calling you to step into a new way of being you.

The Lord will bring you safely through. He will enable you to let go and grow. He wants you to live a righteous and holy life. Food addiction is no match for the wonderful life God has for you.

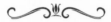

God is calling you to step into a new way of being you.

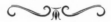

Freedom Reflection

For today's writing, create two columns. Label the left column "Old Nature" and the right column "New Nature." List character traits that need to go on the left and what you hope to replace them with on the right.

Day 35

Opportunities for God's Love and Growth

If we confess our sins to him, he is faithful and just to forgive us our sins and to cleanse us from all wickedness.

1 JOHN 1:9

You don't have to make a big deal about your sins. You just need to bring them to God, ask for forgiveness, seek His guidance, and then move on with life. Don't sit around beating yourself up because of your imperfections or mistakes. Don't get caught up in the destructive cycle of blaming and shaming yourself. It is time to see your journey through God's eyes.

If you notice an area in your life that needs help, you should view it as God does: an opportunity to transform that area through His love. Our admission of each failure or sin provides a chance to invite God in for healing and hope. Each confession of our own shortcomings leads to an even greater testimony of

God's healing grace. Rest assured that every area of refinement is just another part of your story that God will use for His greater good. Today, I encourage you to welcome the deepening of your faith in the confession of your own shortcomings.

Freedom Reflection

What do you need to ask forgiveness for from our loving God? Besides food abuse, what are you shaming yourself about today? What weakness is He working to redeem in your life? How can this help others who are on a similar journey?

Day 36

Let God's Peace Be Your Sedative

Don't worry about anything; instead, pray about everything.
Tell God what you need, and thank him for all he has done.
Then you will experience God's peace, which exceeds
anything we can understand. His peace will guard your
hearts and minds as you live in Christ Jesus.

PHILIPPIANS 4:6–7

Praying about *everything* is so much easier said than done. Today's verse speaks to the truth that prayer is a much better solution for your anxiety than food! Food temporarily calmed your nerves, but now it has taken control of your life. Since you understand that food isn't the lasting solution for your anxiety, I encourage you to give prayer and thanksgiving a try.

Scripture says that you will experience God's peace, which will guard your heart and mind. My friend, *peace* is what you

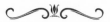

Peace is what you were actually looking for
when you reached for the extra food.

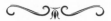

were actually looking for when you reached for the extra food. The need for calming is legitimate, and the discipline of prayer is the truest solution to that need. Lean on God's peace, rather than food, to heal your anxiety and worry, and you will be well on your way to recovery!

Freedom Reflection

This week, practice praying about everything (big and small) and thank God for all He has done. Write down your prayers and keep a gratitude list.

Day 37

God Will Give You Rest!

Then Jesus said, "Come to me, all of you who are weary and carry heavy burdens, and I will give you rest."

MATTHEW 11:28

It probably comes as no surprise that living a frenetic lifestyle can contribute to compulsive overeating. Rushing through your day can leave you unsettled, restless, and more likely to act impulsively with food. It is so easy to let the to-do list of your daily life become more important than your health and well-being. In this day and age, slowing down is not an easy thing to do—but it is still necessary.

Now is the time to modify your lifestyle. Yes, your job, family, and ministry are very important, but you won't have them for long if you don't care for yourself. In your heart, you know that if you are physically, spiritually, and emotionally healthy, your impact on the world will be much greater. I want to encourage you to make caring for yourself a priority, trusting the Lord with the rest of your to-do list. Jesus said, "Come to Me, and I will give you rest." He wants you to cast your cares on Him and trust Him to show you how to live a sane and balanced life.

Freedom Reflection

Take time to think about your schedule and how it impacts your health. How can you make your schedule more balanced? How can you make caring for yourself a priority? Ask the Lord to show you. Write these ideas down to reinforce your commitment to change.

Day 38

My Peace I Leave with You . . .

I am leaving you with a gift—peace of mind and heart.
And the peace I give is a gift the world cannot give.
So don't be troubled or afraid.

JOHN 14:27

If you are honest with yourself, you know your eating addiction is an outward expression of your inward troubles. Your heart and mind have been weighed down with fear and anxiety about relationships, finances, conflicts, and insecurities. You've worried about not being good enough, good-looking enough, wealthy enough, or smart enough. You've probably fallen into the habit of comparing yourself to others, always assuming that you are more flawed than most. You know you are not fully living life in the way God has designed you to live it.

Hiding on the sidelines of life—full of anxiety, fear, and self-judgment—is a miserable existence. Think about His words deeply: "The peace I give is a gift the world cannot give." Jesus left you a gift—not just eternal life after death, but also an eternal *quality* of life. His peace and joy are yours for the taking. He wants you to live life to the fullest!

Freedom Reflection

Make two columns on a page in your journal. Under the first column, list your fears and insecurities. Under the second column, next to each entry from the first column, write these words: *My peace I leave with you.*

Day 39

I Trust in You, Lord

When I am afraid,
I will put my trust in you.
PSALM 56:3

Pay close attention to the honesty and the phrasing of this verse. Instead of denying fear, the psalmist begins his claim of trust by admitting his fear! Being afraid is part of his story, and it is also part of yours. This verse teaches us that we should put our trust in the Lord whenever we feel afraid. Don't get down on yourself about it. *Everyone* is afraid from time to time; it is simply part of being human.

Whenever you become afraid, acknowledge the feeling as normal. Be kind to yourself just as you would to a friend, and reach out to God for help. Say out loud, "I trust You, Lord, even in my fear." Thank Him for being with you and for giving you the strength to face the moment. Remember that God works through other people as well, so make sure to call a friend (or two) and ask them for encouragement through conversation and prayer. It will take some practice to learn to face those difficulties with strength and courage, but it is a much better solution than trying to eat your fears away.

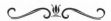

Whenever you become afraid, acknowledge the feeling as normal.

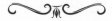

Freedom Reflection

Today, write about a typical experience that causes you to be afraid. Now imagine declaring, "I trust You, Lord!" when faced with that situation. Write about how different it would be to walk through that same scenario with God at your side.

Day 40

Walking Close to the Lord

This is my command—be strong and courageous! Do not be afraid or discouraged. For the Lord your God is with you wherever you go.

JOSHUA 1:9

Do you realize that the God of the universe is walking through life with you—alongside you on the streets, in your home, at your job, and with your family? Do you understand that He is also right there with you in each small step of your recovery?

You are never alone!

When you know the Lord is with you wherever you go, you have no reason to ever be afraid or discouraged. You are loved, safe, and protected, and you have every reason to be strong, courageous, and satisfied in Him. Lasting strength and courage come when you realize the truth of His steadfast presence in your life and learn to rely on Him completely. The further you are from His presence, the more fearful you will become. So walk closely with the Lord and grow in the knowledge of His strength in you.

Freedom Reflection

Do you truly believe God is with you wherever you go? How do you stay aware of Him throughout the day? Make a list of the ways you can increase your awareness of God's steady presence in your life.

Day 41

Dealing with Anger

Don't sin by letting anger control you. Don't let the sun go down while you are still angry, for anger gives a foothold to the devil.

Ephesians 4:26–27

Anger is one of those emotions that so many people have difficulty managing. There is great wisdom in having a plan in place to deal with anger quickly and honestly. If you try to hide anger or hold it inside, there's a good chance you will turn to food to deal with it. If you let yourself rage, you will be so ashamed afterward that you'll likely eat from the embarrassment.

Learning how to use your supports to process your angry feelings is key. Talk to a trusted friend, write in a journal, take a prayer walk, and vent to God. God is a safe place to vent your feelings (just read through Psalms and Lamentations).

Always allow yourself to cool down before voicing your anger with loved ones or coworkers. Stepping aside to think through a matter, to pray, and to receive support can make all the difference in your reactions. These tactics can keep you from hurting anyone, including yourself.

If you're afraid to talk openly about your feelings, you may be passively letting things go while raging on the inside—which is unhealthy behavior and a trigger to overeating. If you struggle with expressing yourself, don't be afraid to get help. Anger can be overwhelming, so don't try to manage it alone.

Freedom Reflection

Spend some time writing in response to the following questions: How do you handle anger? Are you more likely to hide your feelings, or do you let them fly? How has anger gotten you in trouble? Do you see how eating and anger go together? How would you like to improve in this area?

Day 42

Learn to Control Your Anger

You must all be quick to listen, slow to speak,
and slow to get angry.

JAMES 1:19

Learn to listen and think before you react. It's so easy to get angry when you haven't taken the time to listen and think things through. As a person who abuses food, you must understand the importance of keeping your cool. If you let your blood pressure rise, along with cortisol levels (your stress hormones), you're walking into a complete setup for trouble not only with food, but also with the people around you. I encourage you to practice watching over yourself. Notice when anger begins to develop. Learn to say a prayer and take some time to cool down. Find a healthy strategy that helps you manage your feelings, but don't let yourself get out of control.

It takes practice to listen to others (and to yourself) before reacting. Put yourself in another person's shoes and try to understand his or her side of a story. Remember that people make mistakes! Sometimes your acceptance and forgiveness are necessary. Practice listening and accepting the things you can't change. You need this characteristic to recover. Sometimes it is better to have peace than to have everything your way.

Freedom Reflection

What particular issues set you off and make you angry? If you don't know the serenity prayer, it's a good idea to learn it:

God, grant me the serenity to accept the things I cannot change, courage to change the things I can, and wisdom to know the difference.

Write about what it means to accept the things you can't change.

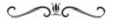

Practice listening and accepting
the things you can't change. You need this
characteristic to recover.

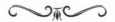

Day 43

Resentment Is a Poison

Love is patient and kind . . . It is not arrogant or rude. It does not insist on its own way; it is not irritable or resentful.

1 CORINTHIANS 13:4–5 ESV

You've probably heard the saying that holding on to resentment is like drinking the very poison you were hoping to give to someone else. Alcoholics Anonymous calls resentment the "number one offender."[5] Keeping hurt and anger unresolved for long periods of time is a dangerous choice. Research shows that there are all kinds of illnesses related to unresolved resentments—and yes, addiction is one of them.

I understand that sometimes it's difficult to let go when your wounds are real and deep. I encourage you to relinquish your resentments, not because whoever hurt you deserves it, but because you do. You deserve to have peace and a mind free of negativity.

Holding on to resentment can trigger you to overeat when you are trying to eat healthy. That kind of negative energy is like rocket fuel for addiction. You must be willing to ask God for help if there are people you simply cannot forgive. The twelve-step programs suggest praying every day for the person you resent, for blessings in their lives—the kind of things you would want for yourself. Try it; maybe you'll find your heart softening, and you might just begin to view those people the way God sees them.

Freedom Reflection

Search your heart today, and every day for three weeks; pray for anyone you resent (You may need to carry a list of people to pray for in this way). Pray for them to be blessed with peace and abundance. Pray for their health and happiness.

Day 44

Forgiveness Is a Way of Life

---

*Make allowance for each other's faults, and forgive
anyone who offends you. Remember, the Lord forgave you,
so you must forgive others.*

COLOSSIANS 3:13

Forgiveness is fundamental to recovery, and it is helpful to start with remembering how the Lord forgives you. In His eyes, every last one of your trespasses, failures, and shortcomings has been *completely* forgiven. Why? Because every single one of your sins was nailed to the cross. Forgiveness means that God has forgotten them forever. If any part of you still struggles with that truth, go back to the basics of the Gospel and remember everything that was done for you—yes, *you*!

Remember: Jesus forgave the thief hanging next to Him along with all the people who persecuted and crucified Him

In His eyes, every last one
of your trespasses, failures, and shortcomings
has been completely forgiven.

(Luke 23:34). If He forgave them, He most certainly forgives you! And the Bible tells us that He wants you to emulate His lifestyle of forgiveness.

If you believe you are unable to forgive, ask God to help you. It may take some time to get to the place where you can do it. I encourage you to talk to a trusted friend or counselor who can help you carry these burdens and learn to forgive. It may be difficult at first to forgive yourself or those who have hurt you, but I promise, you will quickly discover that you are personally healing by learning to live a lifestyle of forgiveness!

Freedom Reflection

Today, spend some time writing about whom you need to forgive. Take the list you made yesterday of people you resent and pray over it. Write about how your life might change if you were able to fully forgive the people on your list.

Day 45

Don't Hold Grudges

If you forgive those who sin against you, your heavenly Father will forgive you. But if you refuse to forgive others, your Father will not forgive your sins.

MATTHEW 6:14–15

God's command to forgive is serious enough that He put a condition on it: if you refuse to forgive others, then He will not forgive you! Refusing forgiveness is simply not an option. Mark 11:25 explains, "When you are praying, first forgive anyone you are holding a grudge against, so that your Father in heaven will forgive your sins, too." The Bible is resoundingly clear that you are never to harbor unforgiveness. If you have an issue with someone, you should deal with it right away.

Why is God so concerned with forgiveness? Because He loves you and wants you to live in freedom. He knows that if you are unwilling to forgive someone (including yourself), you will be the one truly hurting until it gets resolved. He loves you enough to command you to fix problems with other people *before* you approach Him.

How does this relate to your addiction? Unresolved conflicts lead to inner pain and turmoil, which leads to compulsive eating. The solution is to make forgiveness a daily practice. Let your supports, your family, and your prayer partners help you grow in this area. Remember: God is with you and can give you the strength to forgive others.

Freedom Reflection

Before you pray or worship today, take a moment to consider whether there is anything that needs to be resolved with you and anyone else in your life. If forgiveness is necessary, then begin that process in your heart with God. Write about the struggle, if you think doing so will help.

Day 46

Let the Lord Be Your Comforter

The Lord is close to the brokenhearted;
he rescues those whose spirits are crushed.

PSALM 34:18

You used to turn to food to feel better when you were sad. Somehow, food provided comfort during painful seasons of your life—and that is exactly how you became addicted. The feel-good part of the brain led you to food for a quick, but temporary, fix. But God is so good! As you put the food down and let yourself be honest about the brokenness of life, He will come and provide the true and lasting comfort you need.

The challenge is found in facing your sadness with honesty and transparency, waiting on the Lord, and trusting His love and comfort instead of the temporary satisfaction of food. I know you are here because you have found sadness and grief unbearable. Let's remember together the truth that food isn't truly fixing anything in your life. Its promise is short-lived, and it ends in addiction and disaster. Facing your brokenhearted or sad feelings is a completely normal part of life in a difficult world. I encourage you to run to God for relief in these moments. I promise that He will be there for you in a way that food never will be. He will satisfy the needs of your heart.

Freedom Reflection

Write down some examples of times you have used food for comfort when you were feeling down. How did the food make you feel? Then write examples of times you experienced sadness without using food. What difference did you feel? How can you better learn to trust God with that sadness?

Day 47

Choosing Gratitude Over Discouragement

Why am I discouraged? Why is my heart so sad? I will put my hope in God! I will praise him again—my Savior and my God!

PSALM 42:11

Whenever you are feeling down, try to be intentional about asking yourself why. Feeling down can actually become a habit. Having negative thoughts about life, yourself, your food abuse, and weight issues can really drag you down.

Why spend your energy thinking about everything wrong with you and the world? That negativity is not doing any practical good in your life. It leads to depression and hopelessness. The psalmist asks himself, "Why am I discouraged? Why is my heart so sad?" Then he answers, "I will put my hope in God! I will praise him again—my Savior and my God!" Yes, there are things to feel down about, but I encourage you to see the world as the psalmist does. No matter the circumstance, you have much to praise God about. Decide to praise God and focus on what is good! I promise that this kind of gratitude will turn your day around.

Freedom Reflection

Make a gratitude list. Each day, for the next seven days, I encourage you to add three things you are thankful for to that list.

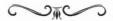

No matter the circumstance,
you have much to praise God about.

Day 48

The Source of All Comfort

All praise to God, the Father of our Lord Jesus Christ. God is our merciful Father and the source of all comfort. He comforts us in all our troubles so that we can comfort others. When they are troubled, we will be able to give them the same comfort God has given us.

2 CORINTHIANS 1:3–4

You have been through a lot in your life. At certain moments the difficulties have overwhelmed you, and you have wondered, *Why me, God?* But if you are honest about your journey, you'll see that you have not only grown, but also become strengthened from many of these overwhelming trials.

God truly does work things out for good. When you are going through tough times, remember that God will see you through. God is merciful and gracious. He is the source of all comfort. You cannot find that comfort in your refrigerator or at the latest restaurant. You will not find inner strength in a trendy weight-loss program or even at the gym. Only He can give you the comfort you really need.

And God's comfort is also strongest when it is shared. As you learn to trust God in this way, you will find your blessings overflowing as He uses you in the lives of others. As you share with others the comfort you have received from God, your strength will also rise—so pass it on!

Freedom Reflection

Reach out to someone else today to see how your personal experience can benefit others. Don't worry if you have not "arrived." You have something to offer people, no matter where you are in your own journey.

How do you imagine God as your comforter? Imagine taking your troubles straight to Him, as if you were sitting right on His lap with His arms wrapped around you. Meditate on that image for a while.

Day 49

The Lord Will Hold You Close

Even if my father and mother abandon me,
the Lord will hold me close.

PSALM 27:10

You may still see food as some sort of friend who has been there through thick and thin. In the past, you have found security and relief from your special treats. Somehow, when no one else felt safe to go to for help, food seemed the safest thing to pick up.

Yes, people can and will hurt you. They will leave you. And they can be cruel. Sometimes it seems much easier to just stick with food. If nothing else, food has temporarily taken the edge off of the pain caused by people in your life!

It can be difficult to even consider giving up this "friend" who has been the only "safe" go-to in your life. Take a moment to focus on the theme of this beautiful verse. Even if the people closest to you abandon you, the Lord will hold you close. And you already know the truth that junk food is not your true friend; it is the furthest thing from a solution. Food has only isolated you, caused you to hate yourself, and made you sick.

Today, hold fast to this truth: you are never alone because the Lord will hold you close.

Freedom Reflection

Meditate today on this scripture and take it by faith. Write down your thoughts about how this applies to your life. Write a goodbye letter to your food addiction. Tell it you are finished with it, and you are now sticking with God.

Day 50

Live Free from Isolation

Father to the fatherless, defender of widows—this is God,
whose dwelling is holy. God places the lonely in families;
he sets the prisoners free and gives them joy.

PSALM 68:5–6

Your addiction creates isolation. You are just beginning to realize the extent to which food has created separation in your life. Overeating has been a lonely ordeal, not something you really want to invite your friends and family to share. And the more you eat, the more isolated you become.

But life can also naturally bring feelings of loneliness. It is possible to feel isolation, even from your closest family members, in ways we have no control over—such as the loss of loved ones, abuse, or divorce. When you turn to food as a solution for your troubles, it only exaggerates the feelings of isolation.

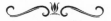

When you turn to food as a solution
for your troubles, it only exaggerates
the feelings of isolation.

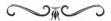

My friend, I want to tell you that there is lasting hope for you. God is a Father to the fatherless and a defender of widows. He places the lonely in loving families. He sets the prisoners free and gives them joy. What hope this world brings! I encourage you to take hold of this hope today.

Freedom Reflection

Write about how God has already been working in your life. Imagine Him providing a place where you are free from the prison of food and surrounded by caring support.

Day 51

Leaving Busyness Behind

But the Lord said to her, "My dear Martha, you are worried and upset over all these details! There is only one thing worth being concerned about. Mary has discovered it, and it will not be taken away from her."

LUKE 10:41–42

Nothing right now is more important than your recovery. Slow down and forget about getting everything done in this moment. Before you try to tackle your to-do list, I encourage you to first sit with the Lord. Make it a daily habit to enjoy some peaceful, sweet time of spiritual refreshment. Make sure to recharge on God's Word and His love, just as you would charge your phone battery. When you spend your days running from task to task without stopping to connect to God, you will set yourself up to crave excess food. You will become physically, emotionally, and spiritually starved.

Mary is a great example for us to follow. Even with all that needed to be done, she sat at the feet of Jesus. My friend, I assure you that there will always be dishes to clean, clients to call, and children to tend, but your spirit simply cannot be ignored. Learn to be disciplined about recharging your spirit each day by spending time with God. He is the source of love and strength in your life.

Freedom Reflection

Write down what tasks you can let go of (or even delegate to someone else) to make room for quiet time with God. Can you live with letting go of everything being done to your standards? In what ways can you protect the time necessary to recharge with God?

Day 52

You Don't Need to Be Perfect

If you wait for perfect conditions, you will never get anything done.
ECCLESIASTES 11:4 TLB

Perfectionism appears in different forms. You may work hard to be sure everything is just right, or you may tolerate nothing but the best in yourself and others. Or you might be stuck waiting and waiting for the best conditions before you act—ignoring that there is no "perfect" time for anything! The truth is, your expectations are never met because *they can never be met*. Compulsive overeating is a common symptom of all kinds of perfectionism. You can use food to either energize you for the unmanageable workload you assume or to numb yourself from the guilt of your procrastination and avoidance.

In recovery, you must change your view completely. It's better to give up worrying about being perfect and just give things a try. Take a chance. Move forward one step at a time. Set fire to your high demands and ridiculous expectations. Don't let the fear of failure or of not being "good enough" keep you from living your life. There is no perfect time to start living; there is no perfect way to begin your recovery. You have to trust God and begin your journey with courage each day!

Freedom Reflection

What have you been holding back in your life for fear of not being good enough? Make a list. How can you let go of the fallacy of perfectionism? What would you like to change?

Day 53

Don't Let Shame Hold You Back!

So don't be too good or too wise! Why destroy yourself?
ECCLESIASTES 7:16 TLB

I'll give it to you straight: you don't have all the answers, and no one expects you to have it all together.

As we have discussed, the guilt from thinking that you are not good enough is a powerful food trigger. Comparing yourself to some gold standard of spiritual or emotional strength is actually damaging to your spirit. It is also destructive to believe that everyone else has it more together than you do. Comparing another person's "outsides" to your "insides" is never healthy. You can never truly know the reality of another person's experience.

Remember that, in God's eyes, you are good enough right now—today, right where you are. What looks to you like a mess in your life, God sees as your beauty. He knows your heart. Yes, He understands your pain and suffering. He knows all about your mistakes, but He only sees the strength, wisdom, and character developing within you. Don't let shame hold you back today. Start right where you are—no matter the mess—and remember that you are a work in progress!

Freedom Reflection

Write what you feel about being "good enough." How do you think God sees you? What does Scripture say about how God sees you?

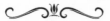

He knows all about your mistakes, but He only sees the strength, wisdom, and character developing within you.

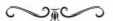

Day 54

Letting Go of Expectations

Love prospers when a fault is forgiven,
but dwelling on it separates close friends.

PROVERBS 17:9

Perfectionism will hurt your relationships. If you are hard on yourself, you will be hard on other people too. When others don't live up to your impossible expectations, you will become disappointed and angry with them. This destructive cycle will cause lasting problems.

God wants you and your loved ones to live free from unreasonable demands. His will is not for any of us to be condemned with perfectionism. Remember, the key to strong relationships is to go easy on yourself and the ones you love.

Approach expectations for yourself and your relationships with the truth of Romans 8:1 in your heart: "There is no condemnation for those who belong to Christ Jesus." Be sure to cherish your loved ones and remember that love covers a multitude of sins. Remember that peace in your relationships is a significant part of the cure for your food addiction.

Freedom Reflection

Are your expectations of others causing difficulty in your relationships? How so? Write about what can you do to remedy this problem in each relationship that comes to mind.

Day 55

Seeking the Approval of Others

Obviously, I'm not trying to win the approval of people,
but of God. If pleasing people were my goal,
I would not be Christ's servant.

GALATIANS 1:10

Be very careful about people-pleasing. There is a difference between loving and caring for people and chasing after their approval. You can spend an enormous amount of time and energy doing things for the approval of others, but that may not be God's plan for your days. Check your motives in each situation to be sure that you are doing God's will. If your motives are self-centered and focused on finding approval, consider walking away from those plans. Take time to think and pray before committing to do what people ask of you. You matter, and your time matters. In order to recover, you need to have boundaries, and you need to say no at times.

Being honest with yourself and living authentically is a part of your new life. If you are acting out of motives that are inauthentic, you will feel that disconnect on the inside—and it can lead you to eat. Remember, you only need to be concerned with pleasing God.

Freedom Reflection

Write about how people-pleasing and chasing the approval of others has been a problem for you. How does this relate to your overeating?

Day 56

Feelings Come and Go;
It's Your Actions That Matter

Remember, it is sin to know what you ought to do
and then not do it.

JAMES 4:17

Motivation doesn't always come when you "feel like it." You may have a list of things you know you need to do for your health, recovery, and spirituality, but the truth is, you probably won't "feel like" eating right and exercising anytime soon. You may think of how nice it would be to have peace, experience God's presence, have the Word deep in your heart and mind— but it's not as easy to get motivated, to wake up early, and to make quiet time.

Sometimes you just have to do the next right thing, take the next small step—regardless of how you feel. Feelings come and go, but your actions lead to change. Make up your mind to follow your food plan every day, exercise three to four times each week, attend two to three recovery meetings each week, and have daily quiet times. Many days, you won't have the motivation to do this; but pray and ask God to help you put one foot in front of the other and follow the plan—especially when you aren't feeling it.

Write out a schedule and follow through on your plan. If you do this consistently for long enough, you will see results, and the motivation will follow!

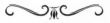

Feelings come and go,
but your actions lead to change.

Freedom Reflection

What's your plan for your recovery? Write down the benefits of following through with that plan (even when you don't feel like it).

Day 57

Overcoming Procrastination
by Asking for Help

Don't put it off; do it now!
Don't rest until you do.
PROVERBS 6:4

Procrastination can be a big problem in recovery. Overeating is a great way to press "pause" on the things you need to do. You might not always want to do what you need to do; some tasks are overwhelming, anxiety-producing, or just plain boring.

You may feel incompetent to complete a task, and instead of asking for help, you simply avoid it for another day. Of course, avoidance causes guilt—and the longer you put off what you need to do, the guiltier you feel. This never-ending cycle leads to food—which you use to drown out the guilty feelings and to keep avoiding what needs to be done.

Remember, your addiction causes feelings of isolation—which is dangerous. You are never alone, even when you are dealing with procrastination. Instead of spinning your wheels and eating yourself into oblivion, ask yourself, *What help do I need? Who can I ask? How can I break this cycle and take one step forward?* God provides helpers through support groups, churches, and many other places. Don't be afraid to reach out for assistance, and don't stay stuck in a cycle of procrastination!

Freedom Reflection

What are your typical areas of procrastination? What do you need to help you get the job done? Make a list of those areas of struggle, then list some strategies you can use to defeat procrastination. Most importantly, identify the people who can encourage you and help hold you accountable in these areas.

Day 58

Always Remain Guarded Against Pride

Pride goes before destruction,
and haughtiness before a fall.

PROVERBS 16:18

You have been clobbered by the repeated loss of control and have learned that your approach doesn't work. It is long past time for you to part ways with the fallacy that you can get healthy on your own. You now understand how much you need to listen to the wisdom of others.

Early in the recovery process, after a few victories, it is tempting to believe that you no longer need the discipline you have learned to stay away from this addiction. When you feel a sense of accomplishment in your recovery, be very careful, because it can be the beginning of a relapse. Today, I want you to embrace the truth that no matter how many victories you have had, your recovery is a journey—and your continued success totally depends on your level of humility.

When you begin to believe you have it all together, that is the very moment you are in real trouble. Even people in long-term recovery understand the nature of addiction, how powerful it is, and how easy it is for someone to be lured back into addictive behavior.

Take a look at Ephesians 4:22: "Throw off your old sinful nature and your former way of life, which is corrupted by lust and deception." The verse doesn't say that your old corrupted nature completely disappears; it must be thrown off, but it is still corrupt. Don't be fooled when you start to feel better: It is when you think you have arrived that you are most at risk!

Freedom Reflection

Have you fallen before because you thought you had it all together? Write about the circumstances of that fall. Make a list of what you need to watch for to keep that from happening again, and pray for the humility to stay the course.

Day 59

The Importance of Being Humble

Humble yourselves before the Lord,
and he will lift you up in honor.

JAMES 4:10

Amazing things are ahead as you begin to get better. You will feel healthier and more energetic, you will look better, and you will start to get positive attention from others for your life change. This can be a source of encouragement, especially when you have felt down in the dumps for so long. But it also can make you feel like running for the hills!

Attention can feel good, but it can also be scary. As the people around you begin to notice the results of your lifestyle change, they will offer their own remarks, both encouraging and hurtful. I want you to remember to *carefully* choose the people with whom you share the details of your journey to recovery.

This is *your* inner journey, and it is far more important than the opinions of others. Your transformation is more about surrendering your food to God than the superficial wonders of losing weight. Be careful to avoid getting hooked on the approval of others. Maintain your humility in the knowledge that, without God and the help of your supports, you would still be a mess. If people compliment you, thank them; but within yourself, give thanks to God. Being humble is easy when you remember that God is doing in you what you could never do on your own.

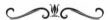

Your transformation is more about surrendering your food to God than the superficial wonders of losing weight.

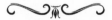

Freedom Reflection

Write about how you have handled attention from others in the past, positive or negative. How has eating been involved?

Day 60

Live in God's Love

Love is patient and kind. Love is not jealous or boastful or proud.
1 Corinthians 13:4

❧

You will discover lasting transformation when you live in God's love and allow the qualities of that love to fill your life. In the past, you have often fallen into the bad habit of self-criticism and condemnation, but now as a recovering person, you know the importance of being patient and kind to yourself and others. Today's verse is a wonderful reminder that you must also guard against the dangerous feelings on the opposite side of the spectrum.

Pride and boastfulness will often show up after you have met a little success. You will be tempted to assume you "know better" than everyone else—or that others simply don't do things the "right way." While it is great to celebrate success, don't allow yourself to become puffed up at the expense of others.

Pride and boastfulness will isolate you from other people. Pay attention to your attitudes and actions through the ups and downs of your healing process. Focus your heart on the characteristics of "living in God's love." As you practice God's way of patience and kindness, a deeper connection to others will strengthen you on your journey to freedom from food addiction!

Freedom Reflection

Write about the people or the circumstances where you find yourself being critical or judgmental most often. How can you learn to practice patience and kindness in those situations? Spend some time praying for God's help in those areas today.

Section Three

Living in Freedom,
One Day at a Time

I am certain that God, who began the good work within you,
will continue his work until it is finally finished.

PHILIPPIANS 1:6

Day 61

Keeping Your "House" Clean

Search me, O God, and know my heart;
test me and know my anxious thoughts.

PSALM 139:23

In most twelve-step recovery programs, practicing daily "check-ins," or "inventories," helps keep what is called a "clean house." Keeping a clean house is a great metaphor for taking notice of your emotional, spiritual, and physical condition. Think about how important it is to maintain where you live. Each day dust builds up, papers collect, clothing piles up, and before you know it, it's time to clean again. It is necessary to keep up with your housecleaning each day, because letting it go ends up leaving you with a huge job!

It is the same with your emotional, spiritual, and physical condition. You will save a lot of heartache and be at higher odds for stable recovery if you practice dealing with any emotional or spiritual issues each day as they arise. If you are feeling down, depressed, angry, or have an unresolved conflict, find your way through it before you end up so low that you are tempted to reach for a pint of ice cream. Remember that these unresolved issues and the related emotional discomforts are fuel for food abuse.

Freedom Reflection

Take time today to write about what has been going on—the good, the bad, and the ugly. You can write it as a letter to God, if you want. However you choose to express yourself on paper, don't avoid this important step in keeping a "clean house."

Day 62

Turn Your Cares Over to God

Give all your worries and cares to God, for he cares about you.
1 Peter 5:7

Each day, as you take time to journal or reflect, pay close attention to any worries or cares that are bothering you. This is an important part of keeping a "clean house." You don't want these worries and cares to pile up and become unmanageable. You may even need to set aside time to intentionally turn your cares over to the Lord. If you have a tendency to become easily worried, you may have to develop scheduled moments throughout the day for reflection and prayer.

Don't be discouraged that you have a tendency to worry. Some of us are just more prone to anxiousness. Instead of judging yourself, take a step into the renewing practice of giving your cares to God. Think of managing your worries like a game

Learning to give your cares to God takes time and practice, but eventually, you will get better at letting things go.

of "hot potato." When worries come your way, focus on passing them back to God immediately. Like everything worthwhile, learning to give your cares to God takes time and practice; but eventually, you will get better at letting things go.

Freedom Reflection

Today, list your worries in a letter to God and then spend some time in quiet prayer. Wait to see what He says back to you. Set aside a few moments each day to practice letting go whenever your worries return.

Day 63

Live One Day at a Time

Don't worry about tomorrow, for tomorrow will bring its own worries. Today's trouble is enough for today.

MATTHEW 6:34

I promise that you will notice dramatic changes when you begin to practice living one day at a time. Try applying this approach in even smaller increments. One hour at a time or even one moment at a time can be life-changing. Thinking in big-picture terms may feel like more than you can handle, but when you break things down into small, manageable steps with short timelines, what feels insurmountable becomes doable.

You can start practicing this approach to life with your food plan—by taking it one meal at a time. The first days are always the most challenging, but each day will get easier. This segmented, one-day-at-a-time or one-hour-at-a-time approach can be helpful at work, in difficult family situations, and when dealing with difficult people. It's a powerful concept. Make sure to remind yourself, *I only have to get through this hour or this day.* And lean on the One who will carry you through these difficult moments by remembering Philippians 4:13: "I can do everything through Christ, who gives me strength."

Freedom Reflection

Write about the areas of your life that could benefit from applying a one-day-at-a-time philosophy. How can this approach help you overcome daily challenges?

Day 64

Overcoming Fear and Avoidance

For God has not given us a spirit of fear and timidity,
but of power, love, and self-discipline.

2 Timothy 1:7

Fear is a big issue for many who struggle with food addiction. Food became your way to cope with fear. Instead of facing the scary issues in your life, you hid in a box of cookies for temporary relief. Over time, you learned how to avoid difficult people and situations, but underneath the avoidance was fear and timidity.

Food was always your coping strategy, but now you understand that you have never built the necessary skills to manage difficult situations. My friend, it is time to learn how to face troubles head-on. Whenever you notice fear and timidity in your daily life, do not let them gain any ground.

Take action! Begin by praying and asking the Lord to help you face whatever you are avoiding. Reaching out to your supports can also be a great help to overcome fear. Today, spend some time meditating on 2 Timothy 1:7 and remembering how God has given you the power, love, and self-discipline to confront your problems head-on.

Freedom Reflection

Is there anything in particular that you tend to avoid because of fear and timidity? Write down a list of these situations and pray over them in the coming week. Also, write a list of the people in your life who can help you face your fears.

Day 65

When You Feel Down, Call Out to God

The Lord hears his people when they call to him for help.
He rescues them from all their troubles.

PSALM 34:17

You know that, on some days, you're just going to feel down. It's not an unusual experience early in your recovery, especially as those feelings that were numbed by food come flooding into your life each day. You may even feel depressed at times. Then, of course, there are the real reasons to feel sad, such as loss, broken relationships, or loneliness. Whether you are feeling brokenhearted, angry, or hurt, take time to listen to your heart. Try to discern what you *truly* need whenever you turn to the fridge. Don't judge your feelings. Be kind to yourself and open your heart to God in those moments. He wants to be close to you in your brokenness and to meet your every need—but you have to call to Him for help and satisfaction.

Once you have acknowledged your feelings and allowed yourself to be real with God, it is important that you don't live with a depressed state of mind. At the right time, you can intentionally step away from that depressed state by focusing on gratitude and praise. Move on to other things in your life and avoid dwelling on the pain. Remember that God set you free. He longs for you to experience joy and peace!

Practice the strategies that help lift you up when you feel down. Physical exercise, nature, time with a friend, support, therapy, and worship can all be helpful. If nothing seems to work, getting professional help is a good idea for figuring out your next steps.

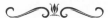

Whether you are feeling brokenhearted, angry, or hurt, take time to listen to your heart.

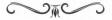

Freedom Reflection

Write down a list of the best depression cures and strategies that you can use when you are feeling down. Make sure not to include food or other addictive behaviors on your list.

Day 66

Find Peace in Relationships

Do all that you can to live in peace with everyone.
ROMANS 12:18

Yes, people can be unreasonable, hurtful, and sometimes even downright abusive. When relationships get tough, it is easy to wonder why you should be the one to make things right. But remember, you have no control over the words and actions of others. You can only manage your responses to them. The principle of doing all you can to live in peace with others begins and ends with you. When you find yourself in conflict with another person, begin by looking at your personal responsibility in that situation, no matter how small, because it will be the catalyst for resolution.

Personal growth comes by learning to look inward first in every relationship. Before you point your finger at others, you should always consider whether there is anything you might be doing, thinking, or feeling that could contribute to conflict or discord. Taking ownership of your own feelings and responses is always the first step toward healing. Interpersonal conflict is a normal part of life, so you need to make a habit of understanding others and praying for God's help in loving them. Remember: irritations, annoyances, and relational discord are fuel for food abuse. Practicing peace toward others will not only save yourself from addiction. That peace will allow you to enjoy healthy connections with people, too.

Freedom Reflection

Revisit your list of people with whom you need to make peace. For each person, write about your responsibility in that conflict. Give these relationships to God today and pray for peace.

Day 67

Weeding Out Your Bitterness and Anger

Get rid of all bitterness, rage, anger, harsh words,
and slander, as well as all types of evil behavior.

Ephesians 4:31

If you've become aware of bitterness and anger in your heart, it's good to be honest about it. Understand that your recovery depends on changing these attitudes. They are dangerous for you and your relationships. God can help you, just as He helps you with your food addiction. You have to confess your bitterness and anger and be willing to allow Him into that space.

As you reflect on your state of being each day, take note when you sense hints of these destructive feelings and attack them immediately with prayer. Just like weeds you see growing in a flower garden, you need to pull them out, lest they spread and choke out the beauty developing in your life. Sometimes you will find that the root of these hurts runs very deep, and you will need the help of others to work through them. Today, I encourage you to embrace the reality that your soul needs to be clear of anger and bitterness so that you can be in the best possible condition for recovery.

Freedom Reflection

As you journal, identify anger and bitterness and make sure to get rid of these on a daily basis. Use support when you need it. Don't let things build!

Day 68

Learn to Crave What Is Pure

---

*Get rid of all evil behavior. Be done with all deceit, hypocrisy,
jealousy, and all unkind speech. Like newborn babies, you
must crave pure spiritual milk so that you will grow into a full
experience of salvation. Cry out for this nourishment.*

1 PETER 2:1–2

In your daily time of reflection, I encourage you to make
sure you don't have any issues that are outside of God's will for
your life. Remember, you will not feel at peace when you are
outside of God's will. For example: If you are living a deceitful
life, you will be weighed down with guilt from knowing you
are not truthful. If you are jealous of others or what they have,
you will feel empty. If you are pretending to be godly while
living otherwise, it will only leave your soul in knots. Any
internal discord is fuel for food abuse, so it all has to go!

If you notice these attitudes and behaviors, bring them before God and call your supports for help. Scripture teaches that you should crave purity if you want to grow into the full experience of salvation. The Lord is in the process of cleansing you daily from all that separates you from His will. He wants you to be filled with the kind of nourishment that will properly grow your soul and spirit. It is not just a step in your recovery; it is essential to living your life to the fullest.

Freedom Reflection

Do you identify with having deceit, hypocrisy, jealousy, and unkind speech in your life? Are there any particular areas you need help with? What do you think pure spiritual milk is, and how does that help?

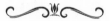

The Lord wants you to be
filled with the kind of nourishment that will
properly grow your soul and spirit.

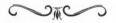

Day 69

The Importance of Building Character

We can rejoice, too, when we run into problems and trials, for we know that they help us develop endurance. And endurance develops strength of character, and character strengthens our confident hope of salvation. And this hope will not lead to disappointment. For we know how dearly God loves us, because he has given us the Holy Spirit to fill our hearts with his love.

ROMANS 5:3–5

Instead of running from your problems the way you did in the days of your food addiction, you are now learning to face those problems with God's grace. You didn't think about the strength of your character until you put down excess food and realized how spiritually sick you had become from your addiction. It is important to face the truth that your unhealthy dependence on food has actually stunted your growth as a person.

It is time to get back on track by committing to developing the strength of your character. It may feel difficult to give up on childish reactions and to meet challenges head-on, but with each step, you are now becoming who the Lord created you to be. Each time you face a tough decision squarely and make the right choice, it strengthens your resolve and maturity. Understand that God is walking alongside you as you grow in character and maturity. That newly developed strength will be necessary for the great blessings God has planned for you, so be open to the rebuilding that God is doing in your inner life. Remember: He loves you!

Freedom Reflection

What are some of the ways in which you can identify your own immaturity? How would it be different if you were mature in those areas? What steps can you take to change those areas of your life?

Day 70

Fix Your Mind on What Is Good

And now, dear brothers and sisters, one final thing. Fix your thoughts on what is true, and honorable, and right, and pure, and lovely, and admirable. Think about things that are excellent and worthy of praise. Keep putting into practice all you learned and received from me—everything you heard from me and saw me doing. Then the God of peace will be with you.

PHILIPPIANS 4:8–9

In the struggles and the busyness of everyday life, staying focused on the Lord is certainly a challenge. Be disciplined to make time every day to pray and reflect on God and His goodness. This is the work of the heart and the path to true recovery and freedom. Today, I encourage you to take your eyes off of food, the scale, the diets, and the insane weight goals. Then, fix your mind on what is true and honorable, right and pure, lovely and admirable.

If you really want to live in peace, start focusing on the health of your soul. Don't be caught up in the insanity and busyness of the world, and don't be overwhelmed by discouragement when it comes your way. Fixing your thoughts on the heart of God is a choice you have to keep making. I hope you will put one foot in front of the other today: Practice, practice, and practice some more, and you will find your peace.

Freedom Reflection

Beyond the practical steps of following a food plan and using supports, what are some actions you can take toward recovery today? Spend some time considering Philippians 4:8. What does it mean to you to "practice all you learned and received"? How can you apply this to your daily life?

Day 71

Seek Peace and Hold Onto It!

Search for peace, and work to maintain it.
PSALM 34:14

⌇

You may believe that there is something wrong because you don't feel peace much of the time. I am here to tell you that you are actually in good company. Don't be discouraged for feeling that way. The good news is, peace is a gift that was promised to you!

Finding peace and hanging on to it are key steps in your journey to be free from food abuse, so make it your business to achieve them. The psalmist in today's verse is giving you an active command, and his instruction reflects the truth that peace won't just show up and knock on your front door. You have to go looking for it!

So what does it mean to seek and pursue peace? I believe that we are to begin each day by making peace our goal—to keep this endeavor for peace prioritized above other things that may be going on in your life. Make it a discipline to consider how every action and decision will affect your peace. Ask questions like these. *How important is each choice in light of my emotional well-being? How will it impact my spiritual life? How will this affect my personal health or my recovery from food addiction?* You need to ask such questions if you value peace in your life.

Freedom Reflection

What are the primary challenges to your peace? How can learning to ask these questions help?

Day 72

Finding God in the Stillness

Be still, and know that I am God!
PSALM 46:10

❦

Finding a way to calm yourself will make a big difference in your ability to remain free from food abuse. Before you began this journey, food was your sedative. Memorize this verse from the Psalms and repeat it to yourself several times each day. When you become disquieted, tell yourself, "Be still." Repeat this phrase over and over as a prayer, and breathe in the message until you feel the inner quiet. "Know that He is God"—not some impersonal god, but the God who loves you. Remember that you can "be still" *because* "He is God." It should take some pressure off to understand that you are not God and you do not have to be! You can hand your troubles over to Him.

Remember that you can "be still" *because* "He is God."

Today, if you have more to do than you can possibly manage, be still and know that He is God. If there is someone you love dealing with an illness, be still and know that He is God. If you have more bills than money to pay them, be still and know that He is God. If you practice living this way, day after day, you will find your need for excess food and junk food diminishing.

Freedom Reflection

Today, begin to practice this beautiful verse from the Psalms as your prayer: "Be still and know that He is God." How can this prayer change your perspective on life?

Day 73

Meditate on God's Word

They delight in the law of the Lord, meditating on it day and night. They are like trees planted along the riverbank, bearing fruit each season. Their leaves never wither, and they prosper in all they do.

PSALM 1:2–3

In recovery groups, it is said that food addiction is a physical and emotional problem with a *spiritual* solution. Prayer and meditation, along with a food plan and support, are all keys to long-term freedom from food abuse. Taking time to bask in God's presence can fill the void in your life. Reading and meditating on God's Word provides wisdom and guidance for every area of living.

You will discover the peace and wisdom gained through meditating will be available in every situation you encounter.

When you are faced with difficulties, God's Word will guide you. As your mind is no longer fixated on food, negative body thoughts, and harmful self-talk, you will become aware that God is changing you into the person you always hoped to be. Today, I challenge you to meditate on God's love and let His Word fill your mind and heart.

Freedom Reflection

Try this meditation activity. Take a short passage or even one verse and really take it in. Think about what you read. Think about how it applies to your life. What does it mean to you? How do you relate to it? Let the meaning go down deep into your heart until you are blessed by it. Try to remember what you meditated on throughout the day. Keep it simple.

Day 74

God Will Meet You Right Where You Are

Draw near to God and He will draw near to you.
JAMES 4:8 NASB

∽

Do you ever wonder if God actually cares about your struggle with food? Maybe you feel that it's your job to fix your food addiction *before* you go to Him. You might feel distant from God because someone did something hurtful to you in His name, but in your heart, you know your addiction is a God-sized problem. You know you can't do this without divine help, yet it seems you can find a hundred reasons to feel separated from God. Doubts and questions come and go and are a normal part of faith, but don't let them take root in your life and make you feel alone.

When you are feeling discouraged, reach out to God no matter where you are or how you are feeling. Scripture says that if you come close to God, He will come close to you. Put aside your questioning and doubting for now. You can always come back to it, but give God a chance. How will you ever know if God could help unless you try to open up to His care? Intimacy and trust may be difficult for you, but God is a safe haven. He can handle your questions and doubts! God's love is never failing. Trust His Word and allow Him to draw close to you today . . . right where you are.

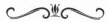

Intimacy and trust may be difficult for you, but God is a safe haven.

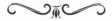

Freedom Reflection

Make a list of the things that are blocking you from drawing near to God. For today, try to let go of the reasons and give God a try.

Day 75

You Are Wonderfully Made

---

*You made all the delicate, inner parts of my body and knit me
together in my mother's womb. Thank you for making me so
wonderfully complex! Your workmanship is marvelous—how well I
know it. You watched me as I was being formed in utter seclusion,
as I was woven together in the dark of the womb.*

PSALM 139:13-15

During these years of overeating, you have wrestled with
negative feelings about your body. You have stared into the
mirror and dealt harshly with yourself over each little perceived
imperfection. Isaiah 64:8 declares, "And yet, O Lord, you are our
Father. We are the clay, and you are the potter. We all are formed
by your hand." Consider the truth that you are complaining about
God's craftsmanship when you beat yourself up before that mirror.
To be more direct: The Creator of the universe designed you, and
now you have decided that He didn't do a good enough job?

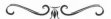

It is time to start appreciating
the beauty of God's creation in you.

I challenge you today to walk away from your personal body-shaming and negative self-talk. It is time to start appreciating the beauty of God's creation in you. When you can see through God's eyes how delighted He is with you, and when you can recognize your own beauty, you will start to recover on the inside. It is time to begin seeing yourself through God's eyes. Stop picking on your imperfections. Look for the magnificence of His awesome work in you!

Freedom Reflection

Meditate on the truth that you are fearfully and wonderfully made. For the next few days, write about what is good and beautiful about you. You are creating a new way of thinking about yourself, so even if you begin with one or two things, that is okay!

Day 76

Love the Lord with All Your Heart

You must not have any other god but me.
DEUTERONOMY 5:7

When you were turning to food for comfort, for friendship, for a lift when you were down, it was as if you were turning to a false god. The Bible tells us that God is jealous, and He does not want us to have any other gods except Him. Why is God "jealous"? Because He wants what is best for you! You already understand from your experience with food that false gods may seem appealing, but eventually they lead to illness, hopelessness, and addiction.

Today, reach for the Lord and His strength. Admit that food and the scale have been false gods in your life. Make up your mind to follow Him, and realize that when you are tempted to abuse food and your body, it is basically no different than returning to a strange god. There is real power in understanding your addiction on a spiritual level in this way. Put *nothing* before God. As Jesus commanded in Matthew 22:37, "Love the Lord your God with all your heart, all your soul, and all your mind."

Freedom Reflection

What is the difference between following and obeying God the Father and following and obeying the "food" god? In what ways have you allowed food and the scale to play the role of a god in your life? Describe the difference in your life when you are following God and when you are following your false god.

Day 77

Embrace the Freedom God Offers You

If the Son sets you free, you are truly free.
JOHN 8:36

◦⌒◦

It requires faith to believe that the Son of God has set you free. If you are a believer, then Jesus died on the cross to bring you into a life of freedom. Imagine the chains of your food addiction being cut away. Envision yourself leaving that place of bondage and beginning a new life with no more binges, no more shame and guilt, no more hiding or lying. If you believe in Jesus, then this is the life He wants you to embrace.

The only work left is for you to take hold of this freedom. The chains of addiction are broken, and your prison door has been unlocked, but you have to take the footsteps past the threshold and into the open air of freedom. You have become so used to living in your addiction that you may not even know what to do next. Life outside of food abuse and self-hate seems foreign to you. Trust God today by simply taking the next right step. Don't worry about how strange it feels. Put the healthy food plan together and follow it as if you could actually do it. Learn to lean into your supports when you run into trouble. Act as if you are free, because you truly are. Behave like a free person until you actually believe it. God's Word doesn't lie, but you need to take the first steps and trust Him to be there when you need help. He will satisfy your every need.

Freedom Reflection

What does freedom look and feel like to you? In what ways have you been hesitant to embrace God's freedom in your life?

Day 78

A Way Out of Temptation

The temptations in your life are no different from what others experience. And God is faithful. He will not allow the temptation to be more than you can stand. When you are tempted, he will show you a way out so that you can endure.

1 CORINTHIANS 10:13

Temptation will show up, so it is important to prepare for it by having a plan of action. Learn to think ahead in all situations so you can be ready. At times, you may feel cravings and temptation so strongly that you can't imagine getting through it; but if you are prepared to seek the Lord for a way out, and you stick with your plan, you will be able to endure until the cravings pass.

Remember, if you are eating a healthy food plan, you will not starve between meals even if you see food that you want.

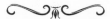

Resolve to stick to your plan regardless of your feelings and thoughts.

Resolve to stick to your plan, regardless of your feelings and thoughts. Cravings are just feelings; they will come and go! God is faithful, and He will help you through these moments. He will always be present and give you the strength you need to follow your plan.

Freedom Reflection

In what ways has God already begun to show you how to avoid temptation? Make a list of things you have learned.

Day 79

The Secret of Contentment

I know how to live on almost nothing or with everything.
I have learned the secret of living in every situation, whether it is
with a full stomach or empty, with plenty or little.

Philippians 4:12

Learn to be content in all circumstances. I understand that it is much easier to be content when everything is going well, when everyone is healthy, the bills are paid, and the sun is shining. Unfortunately, life isn't always so sweet. Life is naturally full of ups and downs, good days and bad days, sunshine and rain. You will have days when everything is going your way and days when it seems as though nothing is right.

Make it your business to see how the difficult days are simply opportunities to grow. Try to understand the troubles you encounter as character-building moments. Don't always assume when you are having difficulty that you have lost God's favor or that He is not hearing your prayers. He is working behind the scenes in every situation, even when you cannot see Him. Learn to practice praising God no matter your circumstances. Choose to be grateful in all things, and you will find yourself content no matter what happens. Before you know it, you may even find yourself dancing in the rain on those gray days instead of bingeing on cookies and ice cream!

Freedom Reflection

Take out the gratitude list I asked you to create in section two of this devotional. Go back and read through the things in your life you are grateful for. How does looking back on this list make you more content with your life?

Day 80

God Is Your Refuge

God is our refuge and strength,
an ever-present help in trouble.
PSALM 46:1 NIV

Troubles are a normal part of life. In the past, you have hidden from your troubles in excess food—yet each time you have turned to food for relief, you have lost an opportunity to grow. Life can seem like an obstacle course at times, but these obstacles make you a stronger person. And when you learn to look to God as your refuge and strength, you will find He is truly ever-present.

Learn to bring your troubles before the Lord in prayer. Allow Him to be the source of your strength when you are faced with trials. Learn to move toward those troubles under the shield of His loving and protective care. As you practice leaning on

Him, you will notice yourself growing stronger. Running to food for comfort in the face of every challenge has made you sick. Moving forward in this journey toward freedom means that you look to the Lord for refuge and know that He will give you the strength to face your every battle.

Freedom Reflection

List all of the ways you have allowed food to be a refuge in your life. How can you continue to make the Lord your refuge instead?

Day 81

God's Mercy Is New Every Day

The faithful love of the Lord never ends!
His mercies never cease. Great is his faithfulness;
his mercies begin afresh each morning.

LAMENTATIONS 3:22–23

Every day is a new day full of new opportunities to move toward freedom from food abuse. Whatever happened yesterday is in the past. In the moments you feel weary of your fight or down about a past failure, the greatest news is that God's mercy never ends. His mercy arrives new, each and every day.

What a wonderful blessing it is to have a chance for a fresh start every day. Yesterday doesn't count against you. God wants you to accept this great gift of a new day and try again. He wants you to try and try until you can take steps toward freedom without falling. If you have walked ten feet and fallen down, wipe off the dust, get up, and keep walking. And remember: you still walked ten feet closer to freedom! You are learning, and every step you take counts. You are growing with each new day. God's mercy and unfailing love is there in all the other aspects of your recovery as well. Whether it is the cravings, the character issues, fear, anger, insecurity, or procrastination, each day brings a new chance and the Lord's unfailing love to help. So don't fret about the past. Embrace every morning as a new beginning.

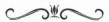

God's mercy and unfailing love is there in all the other aspects of your recovery as well.

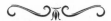

Freedom Reflection

In what area of your journey do you need to practice accepting God's daily mercy? What have you been doing about that area? How can learning to embrace the mercy of a new day change your situation?

Day 82

God's Love Is the Foundation

Keep yourselves in God's love as you wait for the mercy of our Lord Jesus Christ to bring you to eternal life.

JUDE 21 NIV

∽

The love of God is the only foundation you need to recover and heal from addiction. Why? Because your actual transformation depends on His love. When you experience God's love, you are filled with a deep and lasting satisfaction. You once needed to use food to fill the emptiness of your soul, but now that void is filled by the divine love you find in Him. Today, you need to remember that God's love is the key to a deep, contented recovery.

Just a cursory reading of the Bible will tell you that it is part of the human condition to constantly forget about God's love. But if you keep your heart open, you will notice Him continually pursuing you with that love. There is a place in your heart that only He can fill. Your addiction recovery has shown you that anything else you use to fill that void will only leave you broken and longing for more. A huge part of your journey is learning *how* to let God love you—because in His love, the longings will end, and you will experience true satisfaction.

Freedom Reflection

Do you truly know God's love? Write about how you experience His love and presence. What keeps you from knowing and experiencing the love of God?

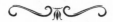

God's love is the key to a deep,
contented recovery.

Day 83

Dependence on God's Power Is Key to Success

Humble yourselves under the mighty power of God,
and at the right time he will lift you up in honor. Give all your
worries and cares to God, for he cares about you. Stay alert!
Watch out for your great enemy, the devil. He prowls around
like a roaring lion, looking for someone to devour.

1 PETER 5:6–8

It is so important for you to stay humble on your journey toward freedom from addiction. Never allow yourself to believe you have it made. Always be on guard against the enemy that is seeking to tear you down, especially in the moments when you believe you have it all together. Your ability to stay the course depends on your spiritual condition. Your reliance on God is the way to long-term success.

Be on guard when you begin to find success in your recovery. When you are doing well, be thankful and know that it is a gift from God. It is He who lifts the obsession and enables you to live sanely with food and your weight. But remain vigilant in your boundaries toward food. Do not become lazy about sticking to your healthy plan. Be firm in your resolve, and keep the door closed to anything that will take you off course. Lean on God to give you strength, and give Him credit for your move toward freedom. Trust Him to protect you from the enemy—especially when things seem to be going well.

Freedom Reflection

At what times are you vulnerable for the enemy to come and take you down? How can you learn to lean on God in those moments?

Day 84

Learn from Your Mistakes

Though they stumble, they will never fall,
for the Lord holds them by the hand.

PSALM 37:24

Stumbling is part of the experience for *everyone* on the road to freedom from food abuse. Maybe you have messed up by taking liberties with food, had seconds when you knew better, or even eaten something outside of your healthy plan. Don't let these mistakes send you back to square one. Allow these slip-ups to be teaching moments. Even in instances of failure, you can learn to hear the quiet voice of God reminding you to stay strong. Learn to pray for God's help in these moments so that you can avoid them in the future. God and your support system will keep helping you up and keep teaching you until

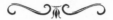

Even in instances of failure, you can learn
to hear the quiet voice of God
reminding you to stay strong.

you learn to walk without falling. Remind yourself there are no failures, just slow successes. Keep on keeping on!

Freedom Reflection

How do you usually handle making mistakes? How can you develop a healthy attitude of learning from your mistakes instead of using them as a reason to fall apart?

Day 85

Don't Be Afraid When You Fall

The godly may trip seven times, but they will get up again.
PROVERBS 24:16

Like most people wrestling with food issues, you probably feel as though you've tripped more times than you can count. Unhealthy eating really is one of the toughest addictive behaviors to give up because it centers on an important part of life. Don't be discouraged when you fall down! When you mess up, don't allow fear to overwhelm you. Remember that God can take our failures and use them for good. There are lessons that we can only learn through trial and error and in the midst of daily mistakes. Whenever you "trip," you will learn where your traps and triggers are and how to lean more on God and your supports for help.

There is power in the lessons you are learning, even when you trip and fall—so don't be afraid to get up and move forward. If this journey toward freedom from food addiction also teaches you to love and depend on God, your blessings will be doubled!

Freedom Reflection

What have you learned about how to recover when you trip and fall? How can fear block you from learning from your mistakes?

Day 86

Never Give Up

Let's not get tired of doing what is good. At just the right time we will reap a harvest of blessing if we don't give up.

GALATIANS 6:9

Whatever you do today, don't give up. The journey to freedom can feel impossible at times for *everyone*. You will likely struggle as you learn to live without food fixes, to manage the new feelings that will surface, and to develop new coping strategies that don't include eating.

Every step in the early months of recovery can feel like a battle. Whatever you do, don't quit—just keep taking those small steps forward. Eventually, you will find it easier to stick with your plan. Your taste buds will change, and you will learn to enjoy healthier food options. You eventually will strengthen your ability to manage emotional triggers, and you will face life head-on with God holding your hand. Yes, all of this takes time and intention—but I promise that if you keep at it, you will arrive at that place of freedom. Today, remember this one important truth: None of this can happen if you quit!

Freedom Reflection

List some of the circumstances that can make you feel like quitting. How can you keep yourself from giving in to the temptation to give up? Spend some time praying for the courage to keep moving forward in those moments.

Day 87

Two Are Better Than One

Two people are better off than one, for they can help each other succeed. If one person falls, the other can reach out and help. But someone who falls alone is in real trouble.

ECCLESIASTES 4:9–10

Let me remind you that learning to ask for help, allowing people to be close to you, and admitting all the ways you really struggle can be a challenge. We really need other people if we are going to survive this journey toward freedom. Yes, it can be embarrassing to be transparent with another person about your struggles. It is not easy to share your obsession with the scale, your negative body image, your fixation on food, or your fears about losing control again. But your new commitment to living free from food abuse requires you to let people help you.

You were not designed to do this on your own. People understand where you are, and they want to help. If you are still holding back from reaching out, it's time to push past the discomfort and take the leap. Start with small increments of trust-building to help you feel comfortable. It may take several attempts to find the right supports, but don't give up! Keep trying until you build a strong support system. As you connect to others, celebrate your successes with them! Don't try to do this on your own, my friend. Together is always better.

Freedom Reflection

If you have not yet begun to build your supports, it's time to get started. In fact, I encourage you to begin today! Make a phone call to someone in recovery. Create a support circle of at least five people.

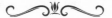

We really need other people if we are going to survive this journey toward freedom.

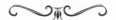

Day 88

Shine a Light for Others

No one lights a lamp and then covers it with a bowl
or hides it under a bed. A lamp is placed on a stand,
where its light can be seen by all who enter the house.

LUKE 8:16

As you make progress in your recovery, one of the best ways to solidify the work happening in you is to share it with others. Don't worry about having it all together; whatever you have learned in your journey will be useful to others. Telling others your story will only strengthen your confidence and your progress toward freedom. Don't listen to the inner voice that will try to discourage you from reaching out to others. Even if you have one good day under your belt, it means that you have learned one thing that is helping you toward your goal. And that means you have something worthy to share.

Because of your addiction, you've hidden in isolation for a long time, hoping no one would see you. It takes courage to come out of that hiding place and share the work that God is doing. Where two or more are gathered, God is also there. He will be with you as you let your light shine. The world desperately needs to know the hope that He is bringing into your life. You need to bear witness to the truth that He can heal food addiction. God wants you to bring His light to the world!

Freedom Reflection

Today, reach out and find a way to help someone. Share something you learned at a meeting or group session with someone who may need it.

Day 89

God Has a Good Plan for You

"For I know the plans I have for you," says the Lord.
"They are plans for good and not for disaster,
to give you a future and a hope."

—JEREMIAH 29:11

God's ultimate plan for you is a life of freedom. He did *not* call you to spend your days in bondage to food addiction. He called you to a peaceful and abundant life. He created you for joy. After spending years in food abuse, you might have wondered if you were going to be stuck in this mess forever. You may have become hopeless. But now it is time to trust God's intentions for your life.

Get it out of your mind that a life of food abuse is an option for you. It is not! Decide today to trust that your future will be hopeful and that you will live the good life God has planned for you. Decide to believe God regardless of the history that got you into your addiction. You are on a new path now. Trust the Lord's design for your life!

Freedom Reflection

What is the future that you hope for? Start to pray in faith by reflecting on Jeremiah 29:11 in the next few days.

Day 90

God Is Doing a Good Work in You

---

*I am certain that God, who began the good work
within you, will continue his work until it is finally finished
on the day when Christ Jesus returns.*

PHILIPPIANS 1:6

I am so proud of the progress you have made, and I hope that you are encouraged by your steps toward a life of freedom from food addiction. God has begun a good work in you, and He is faithful to complete what He has started. You may struggle on your new path. I know there will be moments when you feel as if you could fall back into your old ways. In those times, I want you to fix your eyes on the new work that God is doing rather than on your past. Keep your eyes on the hope of your promised freedom. If you learn to focus on where you are going, put one foot in front of the other and trust in Him. You will make it!

Practice what you are learning each day. Stick with your eating plan, keeping your food and your life separate. Depend on the Lord for strength, and ask for help from people who understand your struggle. As you take this quest for freedom one day at a time, I pray that the Lord will finish this good work that He has begun in you.

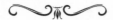

Fix your eyes on the new work that God is doing rather than on your past.

Freedom Reflection

Today, take hold of the truth that God is doing a great work in you. Write about what God wants your life to look like when you are completely healed from food addiction. How will this freedom empower you to live life to the fullest? How will it embolden you to share God's love with others? What will it feel like to be truly satisfied?

ACKNOWLEDGEMENTS

Above all I give thanks to God for setting me free and giving me hope to pass on to others. I am grateful for the people who have gone before me to pave the way to bring helpful tools of recovery to those suffering with disordered eating. Thank you to my clients who have taught me most of what I know by allowing me the gift of walking closely with them in their recovery journeys. To my family and friends for love, patience, prayer, and support in this project—you shaped my vision of the bigger picture for meaningful tools to help people find freedom from overeating and its consequences.

Thank you to my daughters Danielle, Arielle, Jessie, and Jordan for helping in so many ways, providing support, creative ideas, and listening as I wrestled through challenges—your love is greatly motivating. To my friends Sara, Goldie, Marlene, Rachel, Debbie, Margaret, Cheryl S, Marji, Chris, Cheryl K, Virginia and Jennifer as well as several others who are there through thick and thin to listen, pray, and care. I am forever grateful to have you in my life for all things big and small.

Special thanks to Dwight Bain for always believing in and supporting this work and for being a great friend and coach. To

Diane Langberg, I thank you for your love, support, and counsel throughout the years. To Dr. Tim Clinton and AACC, thank you for promoting food addiction treatment for Christians and providing a platform for many people to find help.

Thank you to Matt Litton for coming alongside as a collaborative writer with great writing input and encouragement. Great thanks for all the excellent contributions of the Dexterity Team—Matt West, Heather Howell, and Jocelyn Bailey. Special thanks to Matt West, whose vision, direction, wisdom, and leadership have been invaluable. I also thank Morgan Canclini-Mitchell for helping make the right connections and continuing brand development. For each person mentioned, I thank you for your help and for your heart, love for God and service. I couldn't do this without you!

ENDNOTES

1. Mark Hyman, *Eat Fat, Get Thin: Why the Fat We Eat Is the Key to Sustained Weight Loss and Vibrant Health* (New York: Little, Brown and Company, 2016), 190.

2. "No one can exert cognitive inhibition, willpower, over a biochemical drive that goes on every minute, of every day, of every year." Dr. Robert H. Lustig, pediatric endocrinologist, quoted in "How Sugar Hijacks Your Brain And Makes You Addicted," Healthline.com, http://www.healthline.com/nutrition/how-sugar-makes-you-addicted#section1.

3. All information regarding the Twelve Steps of Overeaters Anonymous can be found at https://oa.org/newcomers/how-do-i-start/program-basics/twelve-steps.

4. "Step One," Alcoholics Anonymous, https://www.aa.org/assets/en_US/en_step1.pdf.

5. "Resentment is the 'number one' offender. It destroys more alcoholics than anything else." From "The 'Number One' Offender,'" Daily Reflections, Alcoholics Anonymous World Services, 1990, https://www.aa.org/pages/en_US/daily-reflection?y=2015&m=04&d=14.

ABOUT THE AUTHOR

Rhona Epstein, Psy.D., C.A.C., is a licensed psychologist, certified addictions counselor, and marriage and family therapist in the Philadelphia area, and the author of *Food Triggers: End Your Cravings, Eat Well, and Live Better*. For more than thirty years, she's led seminars, conferences, and therapeutic workshops to help people overcome food addiction and its underlying issues.

Dr. Rhona received her doctorate in clinical psychology from Chestnut Hill College and her master's degree in counseling psychology from Temple University. Fueled by her own experience and recovery from food addiction, she is passionate about addressing the needs of the whole person (mind, body, and spirit).

Visit Dr. Rhona's web site at DrRhona.com or connect with her on Facebook at @DrRhonaOfficial.

Also available from
Dr. Rhona Epstein

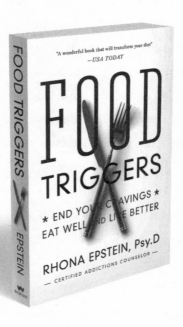

Trade Paper, ISBN: 978-1-6839-7101-6

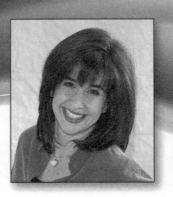
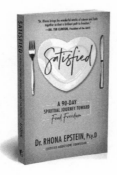